Acute Respiratory Infections

O R M L

OXFORD RESPIRATORY MEDICINE LIBRARY

Acute Respiratory Infections

Edited by

Wei Shen Lim

Consultant Respiratory Physician,
Respiratory Medicine Department,
Nottingham University Hospitals NHS Trust,
City Hospital Campus,
Nottingham, UK

OXFORD

UNIVERSITY PRESS

OXFORD
UNIVERSITY PRESS

Great Clarendon Street, Oxford OX2 6DP
United Kingdom

Oxford University Press is a department of the University of Oxford.
It furthers the University's objective of excellence in research, scholarship,
and education by publishing worldwide. Oxford is a registered trade mark of
Oxford University Press in the UK and in certain other countries

© Oxford University Press 2012

The moral rights of the author(s) have been asserted

First published in 2012

Impression: 1

British Library Cataloguing in Publication Data

Data available

Library of Congress Cataloging in Publication Data

Data available

ISBN 978-0-19-958808-4

Printed in Great Britain by
Ashford Colour Press Ltd., Gosport, Hampshire

Contents

Foreword

Acute respiratory infections remain as big a challenge to human health as they have ever done. At one end of the spectrum they remain one of the most common reasons to consult a GP and at the other end of the spectrum they are an important cause of death. All ages are affected with peak incidences in the very young and very old. The growing human population and especially the growth of the elderly population will increase the numeric importance of such infections.

Against this background new dimensions have been added, many of which are a consequence of human or medical activity. Close contact with animals led to the first outbreak of severe acute respiratory syndrome and has been important for the development and spread of avian and pandemic influenza. Increasing use of immuno-suppressive and immune modulating therapies for an ever expanding list of indications means that infections in those with modified host defences are more and more common. Construction of devices that create aerosols of warm water has opened a route for legionella organisms to enter the lung and cause disease. Crowding together frail individuals in hospital wards and bypassing the normal defences of the lung by endotracheal intubation has facilitated an increase in hospital acquired lung infections.

Antibiotics have been with us now for some 60 years. Despite the importance of bacteria as a cause of acute respiratory infection serious illness and death from such infections remains all too common. Antimicrobial treatment, once thought a panacea, has only relatively recently been recognised to have potentially harmful effects to both the individual and the population as a whole as antibiotic resistance becomes increasingly common. Despite advances viral and fungal infections remain difficult to treat.

Much progress has been made. We have a better understanding than ever before of the array of different microbial pathogens that cause acute respiratory infection. This has facilitated the development of vaccines which are now making an impact on conditions ranging from pertusis to influenza. Clinical studies have led to the development of prediction tools to allow more appropriate stratification of patient care and advances in microbiological techniques have made it easier to detect many causal pathogens. Antimicrobial agents remain the main therapeutic tool at our disposal and the paucity of new molecules currently under development is a concern for the future.

In this setting, a book by acknowledged experts, covering the major areas of acute respiratory infection, concisely written while including the important clinical aspects of these conditions, is a welcome addition, which many interested in or working in this field should find valuable.

Professor Mark Woodhead BSc DM FRCP
Honorary Clinical Professor of Respiratory Medicine
Department of Respiratory Medicine, Manchester Royal Infirmary
Manchester, UK

Symbols and abbreviations

►	Important
AFB	Acid fast bacilli
AIDS	Acquired immune deficiency syndrome
ARDS	Acute respiratory distress syndrome
BAL	Bronchoalveolar lavage
BNF	British National Formulary
BP	Blood pressure
BTS	British Thoracic Society
CAP	Community acquired pneumonia
CFU	Colony forming units
CMV	Cytomegalovirus
CNPA	Chronic necrotising pulmonary aspergillosis
CNS	Central nervous system
COPD	Chronic obstructive pulmonary disease
CPIS	Clinical pulmonary infection score
CRP	C-reactive protein
CVA	cerebrovascular accident
CXR	Chest x-ray
DNA	deoxyribonucleic acid
ESR	Erythrocyte sedimentation rate
ETA	Endotracheal aspirate
FBC	Full blood count
FDA	Food and Drug Administration
FOB	Fibreoptic bronchoscopy
GNEB	Gram-negative enterobacteriaceae
HAP	Hospital-acquired pneumonia
HCAP	Healthcare-associated pneumonia
HIV	Human immunodeficiency virus
HMPV	Human metapneumovirus
HRCT	High resolution computerised tomography
HSCT	Haematopoietic stem cell transplantation
ICU	Intensive care unit

IPA	Invasive pulmonary aspergillosis
IRIS	Immune reconstitution inflammatory syndrome
IVDU	Intravenous drug user
LFT	Liver function test
LDH	Lactate dehydrogenase
LRTI	Lower respiratory tract infection
MDR	Multidrug-resistant
MIC	Minimum inhibitory concentration
MIST	Multicentre Intrapleural Streptokinase Trial
MRSA	Meticillin-resistant *Staphylococcus aureus*
MSM	Men who have sex with men
NHAP	Nursing home-acquired pneumonia
NHS	National Health Service
NICE	National Institute for Health and Clinical Excellence
NPA	Nasopharyngeal aspirate
PCP	*Pneumocystis jirovecii* pneumonia
PCR	Polymerase chain reaction
PCT	Procalcitonin
PCV	Pneumococcal conjugate vaccine
PPV	Pneumococcal polysaccharide vaccine
PSB	Protected specimen brush
PSI	Pneumonia severity index
PUO	Pyrexia of unknown origin
RCT	Randomized controlled trial
RSV	Respiratory syncytial virus
SARS	Severe acute respiratory syndrome
TB	Tuberculosis
TBB	Transbronchial biopsy
TNF	Tumour necrosis factor
U&E	Urea and electrolytes
URTI	Upper respiratory tract infection
VAP	Ventilation-associated pneumonia
VATS	Video assisted thoracoscopic surgery
ZN	Ziehl-Neelsen

Contributors

Thomas Bewick
Clinical Research Fellow,
Nottingham University
Hospitals NHS Trust,
City Hospital Campus,
Nottingham, UK

Claire Blacklock
General Practitioner and
Clinical Researcher
Department of Primary
Health Care Sciences,
University of Oxford
Oxford, UK

Jeremy S. Brown
Reader in Respiratory Infection,
University College London
and Honorary Consultant
in Respiratory Medicine,
University College London
Hospitals,
London, UK

James M. Brown
Clinical Research Fellow,
Department of Thoracic
Medicine, University College
London Hospitals,
London, UK

Morgan Evans
Consultant Physician in
Infectious Diseases,
Ninewalls Hospital,
Dundee, UK

Santiago Ewig
Thoraxzentrum Ruhrgebiet -
Kliniken für Pneumologie und
Infektiologie,
Herne und Bochum,
Germany

Clare Hooper
Pleural Research Registrar,
North Bristol Lung Centre,
Southmead Hospital,
Bristol, UK

Wei Shen Lim
Consultant Respiratory
Physician,
Nottingham University
Hospitals NHS Trust,
City Hospital Campus,
Nottingham, UK

John Macfarlane
Formerly Professor of
Respiratory Medicine,
University of Nottingham
and Consultant Respiratory
Physician,
Nottingham University
Hospitals NHS Trust,
City Hospital Campus,
Nottingham, UK

Nick Maskell
Consultant Respiratory
Physician and Senior Lecturer,
University of Bristol,
Southmead Hospital,
Bristol, UK

John Simpson
Professor of Respiratory
Medicine,
Newcastle University,
Newcastle, UK

**Jonathan S.
Nguyen-Van-Tam**
Foundation Professor of
Health Protection,
University of Nottingham
Medical School and
Honorary Consultant
Regional Epidemiologist
(East Midlands),
UK Health Protection Agency,
Nottingham, UK

Matthew Thompson
Senior Clinical Scientist and
General Practitioner,
Department of Primary
Health Care Sciences,
University of Oxford,
Oxford, UK

Pradhib Venkatesan
Consultant in Infectious
Diseases,
Nottingham University
Hospitals NHS Trust,
City Hospital Campus,
Nottingham, UK

Chapter 1

Acute respiratory infections in primary care

Claire Blacklock and Matthew Thompson

> ## Key points
>
> - Acute respiratory tract infections (RTIs) are common in primary care, comprising approximately 15–20% of all GP consultations
> - 'Safety-netting' and delayed prescribing approaches can help when there is clinical uncertainty, and immediate antibiotics are not indicated
> - Many over the counter treatments for RTIs are available to patients. In children however, the efficacy of some of these is poor
> - Diagnosis of RTIs depends on a focused history and examination, taking account of co-morbidities and other risk factors to guide clinical management
> - Although clinicians often believe their patients expect antibiotics, only a third of patients presenting to their GP with RTIs actually want antibiotics
> - Making a clinical diagnosis of pneumonia without a chest x-ray can be difficult. The key decision is whether an antibiotic is warranted or not.

1.1 Frequency and cost

An estimated 25% of the UK population consult their GP each year because of symptoms of acute respiratory tract infection (RTI). RTIs make up between 15–20% of all GP consultations (and are commoner in children, the elderly, and patients with co-morbid chronic disease). An estimated £15 million is spent annually on treating acute cough alone, and sick leave as a consequence of RTIs is estimated to cost the UK economy a total of £17.3 billion per year.

The incidence of RTIs diagnosed by GPs has decreased considerably over the past decade, which may reflect declining disease incidence or lower consultation rates. Although antibiotics are often still prescribed for RTIs, the rates of prescribing have fallen by up to 50% over the past decade. Moreover, the use of 'delayed prescriptions' means that fewer prescriptions which are issued are taken to pharmacies by patients to be dispensed. Nevertheless 18% of all patients registered with 108 UK GP practices were prescribed an antibiotic for an RTI in 2000.

RTI can cause distressing symptoms that last for days or weeks in many patients, and can recur sometimes several times a year. For patients who are carers, or who provide the main source of income, RTIs can cause difficulties in keeping up with day to day responsibilities. For parents of young children with RTI, they can be a source of considerable anxiety, particularly at night time when sleeping is disturbed.

1.2 **Overall management of RTI**

1.2.1 **Prescribing issues in RTI**
Patients consult a GP with symptoms of RTI for a variety of reasons:
- To confirm the cause of their symptoms
- To seek reassurance that they do not have a more serious illness
- Concerns about how long their symptoms have lasted
- Poor response to over the counter therapies
- To request antibiotics.

There is overwhelming evidence that the majority of RTIs are self-limiting, and most patients will recover without seeking medical help, and without antibiotics. Clinicians often believe their patients expect antibiotics, however recent data showed only 34% of patients presenting to their GP with RTIs actually wanted antibiotics.

Factors shown to increase antibiotic prescribing are:
- Patient factors: expectation of antibiotics
- Clinician factors: perceived patient expectation, feels will build doctor-patient relationship for future consultations, time pressures on prescriber, uncertainty of cause of illness, symptom duration or severity.

1.2.2 **'Safety-netting'**
When immediate treatment with antibiotics is not indicated, use of a 'delayed prescription' may be appropriate, with accompanying instructions on when and how to use it. In primary care, clinicians are not able to monitor patients in the same way as in hospital, so 'safety-netting' is important. This helps to manage clinical uncertainty by empowering patients to know how and when to re-consult.

Box 1.1 Key features of 'safety-netting'
Advise patient regarding:
• Expected natural history of RTI
• Symptoms/signs that may indicate worsening/complications
• What to do if new symptoms arise
• When and where to seek help
• Assess who else is at home.

Antibiotics are associated with side effects, the most common being nausea, vomiting, diarrhoea, rash, plus rarely anaphylaxis. Antibiotics can also interact with other medications such as the contraceptive pill, warfarin, and anticonvulsants.

Antibiotic prescribing is one of the most important factors in promoting resistant strains of bacteria. There is now clear evidence that microbial resistance is associated with:

• Frequent prescribing behaviour
• Use of broad-spectrum antibiotics
• Failure to complete an antibiotic course.

Within primary care, the highest rates of antibiotic prescribing occur for patients with RTIs. In Europe, there is a close correlation between rates of antibiotic prescribing and rates of penicillin resistance in *Streptococcus pneumoniae*. For instance, in the year 2000, rates of pneumococcal resistance were highest in Spain and France, which were also the two countries with the highest penicillin-prescribing rates. England ranked just above Denmark and Germany in resistance rates, but below Belgium and Italy. The lowest resistance rates and prescribing rates were in The Netherlands. In addition, resistance of *H. influenzae* was seen to decrease in parallel with reductions in anti-biotic prescribing in a community in Spain over 10 years.

Another risk associated with antibiotic use is *Clostridium difficile* infection, which is commoner with use of broad-spectrum agents, clindamycin, third-generation cephalosporins, and prolonged use of aminopenicillins. The elderly are at highest risk, with 80% of cases in patients aged >65 years. Other risk factors include hospital admission in the preceding 4 weeks, co-morbidities, use of proton pump inhibitors and residence in a care/nursing home. The incidence of *C. difficile* infection in community settings in the UK is 20–30 per 100,000. Total all-cause 30 day mortality in *C. difficile* infection is 21%.

1.3 **Other treatments**

Additional treatments used for symptomatic relief of RTIs include:

• Antipyretics (e.g. paracetamol, ibuprofen)
• Analgesics – oral or topical (for local pain, e.g. paracetamol, ibuprofen, codeine in adults, benzydamine throat sprays)

- Maintaining sufficient fluid intake and avoiding dehydration (particularly in children)
- Oral steroids - for croup (see below)
- Antitussives (e.g. dextromorphan, codeine derivatives)
- Oral or nasal decongestants (e.g. pseudoephedrine, oxymetazoline)
- Mucolytics (e.g. guaifenesin)
- Natural remedies e.g. honey (some evidence that honey reduces nocturnal cough), nasal saline irrigation.

Other important considerations include:

- Respiratory hygiene measures to reduce transmission to others (especially important in schools, nursing homes, nurseries)
- Patient education/information leaflets (e.g. www.patient.co.uk)— giving information on expected duration, cause, symptomatic medications. They can also help educate patients in self-management and the appropriate use of GP resources
- Smoking status and cessation—a third of cases of community acquired pneumonia in smokers are directly attributable to smoking
- Patients with asthma commonly suffer exacerbation of symptoms with RTI, and may need increased frequency of bronchodilators or sometimes oral steroids. However, there is no evidence that short-acting bronchodilators (e.g. salbutamol) are beneficial in patients without asthma.

A host of over the counter (OTC) preparations for RTIs are available, and include a variety of active ingredients in the form of analgesics, decongestants, antihistamines, antitussives, and mucolytics. Clearly some patients feel relief particularly at night time from cough suppressants (may be due to sedative properties), but overall evidence suggests that in adults the benefit of these medications is inconclusive (no evidence of benefit from antihistamines, and conflicting evidence regarding cough suppressants, mucolytics, and combination preparations). Adverse effects (nausea, vomiting, abdominal pain, dry mouth, headache, dizziness, insomnia) are more frequent than with placebo.

In children there is evidence that OTC preparations do not offer conclusive benefits for RTIs, and may cause adverse events including neuropsychiatric disorders (antihistamines, cough suppressants, mucolytics) and allergy/hypersensitivity reactions (particularly with mucolytics). This has led to several medications being withdrawn or restricted. Overdose from such medications resulted in 230 UK hospital admissions in children under 14 years in 2006/7. Current advice is that children under 6 years should not receive such preparations.

1.4 **Assessment of acute respiratory infections**

The history helps formulate a diagnosis of RTI, identify patients at higher risk of complications, and highlight those who need a face to face assessment. Some patients with uncomplicated RTI can be assessed by telephone and managed safely at home. The history is useful in assessing the overall status of the patient regardless of the site of RTI, and the time-course of illness. Many RTIs have a time course of many days. Key features from the history:

- Presenting symptoms, severity and time-course (systemic features, focal features, previously tried treatments)
- Co-morbidities (esp. COPD and other chronic lung diseases, cardiovascular disease, hepatic/renal disease, dialysis, CVA, neuromuscular disease, immunosuppression, diabetes, malignancies)
- Current medications—can help to further identify co-morbidities and risk factors for complicated RTI (e.g. steroids, inhalers, recent antibiotics)
- Social history (e.g. smoking, self caring or highly dependent, household sick contacts).

Differentiating the various RTIs based on history alone can be difficult as many share common symptoms. In addition, some symptoms found in RTI can also occur in other conditions. For example coryza and fever can occur in children in the early stages of meningococcal disease. Progressive shortness of breath can occur in adults with pneumonia as well as in those with congestive heart failure. Clinically this can be a difficult task—RTIs are extremely common, so it is easy to miss the rare patient with a serious illness. Obtaining an adequate history, eliciting any underlying concerns from patients, parents or carers, and where appropriate offering to see patients face to face to assess them are key to avoiding misdiagnoses. Assessing illness severity at the outset is crucial in the clinical management of RTIs. Clinical signs to take into account when assessing disease severity are given in Table 1.1.

Influenza and respiratory syncytial virus (RSV) are responsible for both upper and lower respiratory tract infections. Specific treatments are available for these infections; please see Chapter 7 for further detail.

Table 1.1 Signs to assess overall severity of illness		
	Adults	**Children**
General/CNS	• Level of fever • Decreased appetite • Change in level of function, confusion (particularly in elderly)	• Level of fever • Difficulty feeding • Less playful, less interested, less reactive during examination, irritable

(Continued)

Table 1.1 (Contd.)		
Respiratory	• Tachypnoea • Decreased oxygen saturations**	• Tachypnoea* • Increased work of breathing (recession—intercostal, subcostal, substernal, nasal flaring, grunting) • Decreased oxygen saturations** • Cyanosis
Cardiovascular/ fluid status	• Raised pulse • Decrease in BP • Decreased urine output	• Raised pulse • Pale/ashen/mottled colour • Prolonged capillary refill • Decreased urine output/no wet nappies

*Tachypnoea (by age):

≥40/min (<1y), ≥35/min (1–2y), ≥30/min (2–5y), ≥25/min (5–12y)

**Oxygen saturations: Decreased O_2 saturation < 92–93% is a red flag for respiratory compromise and (if confirmed on repeat) should prompt a more thorough examination and consideration of pneumonia. A normal O_2 saturation level should not be used to rule out pneumonia, as oxygenation is usually preserved by increasing respiratory effort in the early stages of pneumonia.

In some adults the baseline saturations may already be low (e.g. in patients with COPD), but other adults and children would usually have O_2 saturation over 94%.

1.5 **Upper respiratory tract infections**

Table 1.2 Typical features of common URTIs	
Acute otitis media	• Pain, fever, change in hearing, otorrhoea ± systemic upset. Red, dull, bulging tympanic membrane(s), otorrhoea, unilateral vs. bilateral • Average duration 4 days • Respiratory syncytial virus (RSV), rhinovirus, influenza/parainfluenza virus, *Streptococcus pneumoniae, Haemophilus influenzae, Moraxella catarrhalis* • Complications: recurrent infection, 'glue ear', mastoiditis, intracranial collection
Acute sore throat/ pharyngitis/ tonsillitis	• Sore throat, hoarse voice, odynophagia, fever ± systemic upset (± 'hot-potato voice' in quinsy), injected pharynx, tonsillar enlargement, exudate, tender anterior cervical lympadenopathy • Average duration 7 days • Rhinovirus, influenza/parainfluenza virus, Streptococci group A, C, G etc. • Complications: severe odynophagia (requiring IV fluids), peritonsillar abscess (quinsy), scarlet fever, rheumatic fever

Table 1.2 (Contd.)

Acute rhinosinusitis	• Rhinorrhoea, post-nasal drip, nasal congestion, ± fever, ± tenderness over sinuses • Average duration 2 ½ weeks • Rhinovirus, influenza/parainfluenza virus, *Streptococcus pneumoniae, Haemophilus influenzae, Moraxella catarrhalis* • Complications: chronic sinusitis, venous sinus thrombosis, intracranial collection
Glandular fever	• Injected pharynx, tonsillar enlargement with exudate, fever, malaise, tender lympadenopathy, splenomegaly, hepatic transaminitis • Duration variable: 2–4 weeks to months • Epstein-Barr virus (Monospot test positive, 'atypical lymphocytes') • Complications: persistent fatigue, hepatitis, splenic rupture following trauma, rash with amoxicillin
Mumps	• Painful swollen parotid glands, fever, headache ± painful testicular swelling ± rash • Duration 7–10 days (incubation period 16–18 days, infectious period 6 days before symptoms to 9 days after onset. Outbreaks not uncommon among students, despite vaccination with MMR) • Paramyxovirus (notifiable disease) • Complications: orchitis (25% in post-pubertal males), rarely oophritis, early pregnancy loss, meningitis, pancreatitis, encephalitis, hearing loss
Whooping cough	• Infant: coryza followed by coughing paroxysms with characteristic 'whoop', respiratory distress, vomiting, difficulty feeding • Older children/adults: persistent cough • Duration weeks to months (antibiotics reduce infectivity (5 days after starting antibiotics), but do not alter clinical course) • *Bordetella pertussis* (notifiable disease) • Complications: respiratory distress/dehydration, secondary pneumonia, pressure effects from coughing
Croup	• Coryzal prodrome followed by barking cough, hoarseness, stridor, mainly affects children 6 months–2 years (exclude: foreign body, epiglottitis, bacterial tracheitis) • Steroids useful in management (dexamethasone) • Duration 3 days to 2 weeks • Parainfluenza virus (80%), RSV, adenovirus • Complications: respiratory distress, dehydration

1.6 **Indications for antibiotic treatment of upper RTIs**

1.6.1 **Acute otitis media**

- Children younger than 2 years with bilateral acute otitis media
- Children with acute otitis media and otorrhoea.

This is based on evidence that antibiotics significantly reduce rates of pain and fever at 3–7 days in these groups; by 25% and 36% respectively compared to no antibiotics. In addition, otorrhoea is more likely to be caused by bacterial pathogens and to be more persistent than viral aetiologies.

- Amoxicillin for 5 days (macrolide e.g. clarithromycin, if penicillin allergic).

Box 1.2 **Antibiotic doses in acute otitis media**	
Age	**Amoxicillin dose (from BNF for children 2011)**
Neonate	See BNF for children
1 month–18 years	40mg/kg daily in 3 divided doses (max 1.5mg daily in 3 divided doses)

1.6.2 **Sore throat**

- Patients with acute sore throat when 3 or more Centor criteria are present (see Box 1.4)
- Phenoxymethylpenicillin for 10 days (macrolide, e.g. clarithromycin or erythromycin, if penicillin allergic).

Sinusitis:

- Systemically unwell (and not appropriate to admit)
- Localizing signs of severe sinus infection
- Amoxicillin 1 g tds 7 days in adult (doxycycline or macrolide if penicillin allergic).

Special groups needing referral:

- Patients developing complications of upper RTI (e.g. possible peri-tonsillar abscess, intracranial collection)
- Markedly unwell systemically (e.g. elderly patient with fever and bronchitis who is acutely confused)
- Patients with significant co-morbidities, who are at high risk of decompensation.

Box 1.3 Antibiotic doses in sore throat	
Age	**Phenoxymethylpenicillin dose (from BNF 2011, and BNF for children 2011)**
1 month–1 year	62.5 mg qds (in severe infections increase to 12.5 mg/kg qds)
1–6 years	125 mg qds (in severe infections increase to 12.5 mg/kg qds)
6–12 years	250 mg qds (in severe infections increase to 12.5 mg/kg qds)
12–18 years	500 mg qds (in severe infections increase to 1 g qds)
Adult	500 mg qds (in severe infections increase to 1 g qds)

Box 1.4 Centor Criteria: A predictive tool for Group A beta-haemolytic streptococcal throat infection

- Tonsillar exudate
- Tender anterior cervical lymphadenopathy
- Absence of cough
- History of fever

Interpretation:

≥ 3 criteria indicates a 40–60% likelihood of Group A Streptococcal infection.

< 3 criteria indicates an 80% chance that the patient does not have Group A Streptococcal infection.

Incidence of complications such as peritonsillar abscess and rheumatic fever has not significantly changed with the considerable reduction in antibiotic prescribing over the last decade. Antibiotics cannot be justified in order to prevent these rare complications. For example the number-needed-to-treat to prevent a single case of mastoiditis is estimated to be 2500.

1.7 **Acute lower respiratory tract infections**

The most common lower RTIs are bronchitis, pneumonia, and bronchiolitis. Differentiating the causes of lower RTI can be very difficult in primary care based on clinical features alone. In some adults an urgent chest radiograph can be valuable.

Table 1.3 **Typical features of common LRTIs**	
Acute bronchitis	• Cough, fever, malaise, coryzal symptoms • RSV, rhinovirus, influenza, *Streptococcus pneumoniae*, *Haemophilus influenzae* (a viral pathogen is implicated in the majority of cases) • Average duration 3 weeks • Complications: persistence, worsens stress incontinence, exacerbates COPD
Bronchiolitis	• Typically ≤ 1 year infant with coryzal prodrome, fever, rhinorrhoea, dry wheezy cough • Tachypnoea, recession, widespread fine crackles/high-pitched expiratory wheeze • RSV (80%). Usually seasonal pattern of incidence. • Complications: consider admission if significant respiratory distress or cyanosis, apnoeic episodes, inability to feed, dehydration. Pre-term infants/co-morbid factors important in assessment • Respiratory support and hydration in hospitalized children. • Antibiotics, bronchodilators and steroids are ineffective.
Pneumonia	• See Section 1.7.1 • *Streptococcus pneumoniae* (30–50%), *Haemophilus influenzae* (5–15%), *Staphylococcus aureus*, Legionella, *Mycoplasma pneumoniae*, viral (13%) • Age is a predictor of likely pathogen in children. In younger children a viral pathogen is more likely, in older children *S. pneumoniae*, *Mycoplasma sp.* and *Chlamydophila sp.* are more likely. • Look out for risk factors that predispose to acquisition and/or complications of pneumonia (e.g. aspiration, travel, school outbreak, nursing home resident, diabetes, IVDU, alcohol dependence) • Severity assessment is important as a guide to management • Antibiotics usually required • May need assessment/treatment in secondary care

Cough due to acute bronchitis is often seen as an indication to prescribe antibiotics. However, based on current systematic reviews and NICE guidelines, it may be reasonable to restrict antibiotics to adults aged >65 years with 2 or more (or >80 years with 1 or more) of the following risk factors:

1. Hospitalization in previous year
2. Diabetes
3. Congestive cardiac failure
4. Taking oral steroids

1.7.1 **Diagnosis of pneumonia**

The British Thoracic Society defines community acquired pneumonia (CAP) in adults managed in the community as:

- Symptoms of an acute LRTI (cough plus at least one other)
- New chest signs
- At least one systemic feature (sweating, fever, shivers, myalgia, temperature ≥38°C)
- No other explanation for the illness.

A diagnosis of pneumonia based on clinical features is not very accurate and GPs probably over-diagnose pneumonia. Abnormalities on chest auscultation are highly predictive of antibiotic prescribing by GPs but in reality have low accuracy for diagnosing pneumonia and show poor inter-observer reliability. Tachypnoea, dyspnoea, or pleuritic pain are associated with a radiological diagnosis of pneumonia. In patients with normal vital signs and a normal respiratory tract examination, the presence of CAP is unlikely.

In children, clinical predictors for radiologically-confirmed pneumonia include: fever or a history of fever, breathlessness, reduced breath sounds, crackles, bronchial breathing, chest recession, grunting, tachypnoea and tachycardia. Abdominal pain (referred pain) can also occur.

British Thoracic Society guidelines suggest that bacterial pneumonia should be considered in children ≤ 3 years with fever > 38.5°C, chest recession and a respiratory rate > 50/min. In older children the BTS guidelines recommend that a history of breathlessness is more useful than clinical signs.

A chest X-ray can be useful to confirm the diagnosis or exclude complications (e.g. pleural effusion). In patients with radiological evidence of pneumonia, it is common practice to obtain a follow-up chest X-ray at 6 weeks to ensure the radiological changes have resolved. This is particularly important in patients aged >50 years, in those who smoke, and in those with persisting symptoms or physical signs, due to the risk of underlying malignancy.

1.7.2 **Severity assessment tools**

Severity assessment helps the formulation of an appropriate management plan with the patient which may comprise treatment at home with 'safety-netting' and further review, or referral to secondary care for inpatient assessment.

Several severity assessment scores which are based on the risk of mortality have been developed for adults such as the CRB-65 and CURB-65 scores (see Table 1.4):

CRB-65 1 point for each of:

- Confusion (Abbreviated Mental Test Score ≤ 8/10 or new disorientation in time/place/person)

- Respiratory rate ≤30/min
- Blood pressure ≤90 mmHg systolic or ≤60 mmHg diastolic
- Age ≥65 years.

CURB-65 1 point for each as above plus:

- Urea ≥7 mmol/l.

The CRB-65 and CURB-65 offer very similar performance in predicting mortality in adults. The CRB-65 tool is particularly useful in primary care as it does not rely on laboratory data. BTS Guidelines advise that adults with a CRB-65 score of 1–2 should be considered for hospital referral (particularly score of 2), and that a score of ≥3 should prompt urgent hospital admission.

Table 1.4 Severity assessment of community-acquired pneumonia described as 'CURB-65' with an optional modification to 'CRB-65' (the latter relies on clinical variables alone)

Parameter	Threshold	Points
C = confusion*	present	1
U = blood urea nitrogen	≥7mmol/L	1
R = respiratory rate	≥30/minute	1
B = blood pressure	<90mmHg systolic pressure ≤60mmHg diastolic pressure	1
65 = age (65 years)	≥65 years	1

Classification according to 'CRB-65':
0 points	(1–3% risk of mortality)	= CRB-65 risk class 1 (low severity)
1–2 points	(8–10% risk of mortality)	= CRB-65 risk class 2 (moderate severity)
3–4 points	(30–35% risk of mortality)	= CRB-65 risk class 3 (high severity)

Classification according to 'CURB-65':
0–1 points	(<3% risk of mortality)	= CURB-65 risk class 1 (low severity)
2 points	(9% risk of mortality)	= CURB-65 risk class 2 (moderate severity)
3–5 points	(15–40% risk of mortality)	= CURB-65 risk class 3 (high severity)

* New disorientation in time/ person/ place or Abbreviated Mental Test Score less than 8.

In children with community acquired pneumonia, the following should be considered as indications for hospital admission:

- Respiratory rate >70/min (infants), >50/min (older children)
- Breathlessness
- Significant increased work of breathing including recession, retraction, nasal flaring, grunting
- Intermittent apnoea (infants)
- Oxygen saturations ≤92%, cyanosis (be aware of agitation as a sign of hypoxia)
- Not feeding (infants), dehydration

- Signs suggesting serious infection generally (see Table 1.1)
- Insufficient family support at home.

1.7.3 **Treatment of pneumonia**

GPs prescribe antibiotics to 80% of patients with features of LRTI, even though only a small proportion (<20%) actually have an underlying pneumonia. This mismatch probably reflects a cautious approach and ongoing clinical uncertainty over the accuracy of the diagnosis of pneumonia based on clinical features alone.

The recommended antimicrobial treatment for CAP managed in primary care is:

Adults
1st Line: Amoxicillin 500mg tds for 7 days
Alternatives if penicillin allergic:
Doxycycline 200mg loading dose, then 100 mg daily for 7 days or clarithromycin 500mg bd for 7 days (reduced gastrointestinal intolerance compared to erythromycin).

Children
>5 years of age: 1st Line: Macrolide for 7–10 days (to cover *Mycoplasma sp.*, which is more prevalent in this age group, after *S. pneumoniae*).

<5 years of age: 1st Line: Amoxicillin for 7-10 days (covers most likely pathogens in this age group).

Alternatives: Co-amoxiclav, cefaclor, erythromycin, clarithromycin, azithromycin (all 7–10 days, except azithromycin 3 days).

In children, if there is concern about staphylococcal pneumonia (e.g. following influenza infection), use a macrolide, or flucloxacillin and amoxicillin in combination.

1.7.4 **Follow up**

In all patients with pneumonia, follow-up is important and part of 'safety-netting'. For patients who are treated at home, an initial follow up appointment should be considered within 48 hours to ensure that the diagnosis was correct and that the patient is responding to antibiotics and coping at home. Possible misdiagnoses at an initial re-consultation might include complications of pneumonia itself (e.g. pleural effusion), heart failure, aspiration pneumonia (e.g. patient with compromised swallow after a stroke).

Depending on the clinical situation, other considerations at an initial or later follow up appointment could include:

- Presence of underlying malignancy
- Any evidence of aspiration requiring investigation
- Likelihood of other lung-related diagnosis (e.g. COPD, cystic fibrosis, TB)
- Concordance with childhood immunizations, or indication for adult pneumococcal or influenzal immunizations.

Further reading

Ashworth M., Latinovic R., Charlton J., et al. (2004) Why has antibiotic prescribing for respiratory illness declined in primary care? A longitudinal study using the General Practice Research Database. *Journal of Public Health* **26**(3): 268–274

British Thoracic Society (2002) Guidelines for the Management of Community Acquired Pneumonia in Childhood. *Thorax* **57**(I): i1–i24.

British Thoracic Society (2009 update) Guidelines for the Management of Community Acquired Pneumonia in Adults. *Thorax* **64**(3): iii1–iii55.

Goossens H., Ferech M., Vander Stichele R., et al. (2005) Outpatient antibiotic use in Europe and association with resistance: a cross-national database study. *Lancet* **365**(9459): 579–87

Hopstaken R., Butler C.C., Muris J.W., et al. (2006) Do clinical findings in lower respiratory tract infection help general practitioners prescribe antibiotics appropriately? An observational cohort study in general practice. *Family Practice* **23**: 180–7.

Lim W.S., van der Eerden M.M., Laing R., et al. (2003) Defining community acquired pneumonia severity on presentation to hospital: an international derivation and validation study. *Thorax* **58**: 377–82.

Lynch T., Platt R., Gouin S., Larson C., Patenaude Y. (2004) Can we predict which children with clinically suspected pneumonia will have the presence of focal infiltrates on chest radiographs? *Pediatrics* **133**(3): e186–189.

Margolis P., Gadomski A. (1998) Does this infant have pneumonia? *JAMA* **279**: 308–13.

NICE Clinical Guideline 69 (July 2008) Prescribing of antibiotics for self-limiting respiratory tract infections in adults and children in primary care.

Rovers M., Glasziou P., Appelman C.L., et al. (2006) Antibiotics for acute otitis media: a meta-analysis with individual patient data. *Lancet* **368**: 1429–35.

Sharland M., Kendall H., Yeates D., et al. (2005) Antibiotic prescribing in general practice and hospital admissions for peritonsillar abscess, mastoiditis, and rheumatic fever in children: time trend analysis. *BMJ* **331**: 328–9.

Chapter 2

Community infections in secondary care

Santiago Ewig

Key points

- In patients admitted to hospital with severe acute bronchitis and/or decompensated comorbidity, the need for antibacterial treatment requires careful clinical judgment
- In patients admitted to hospital with acute exacerbations of COPD, respiratory viral pathogens are identified in the majority
- In patients with COPD, there is an association between lung function and the pattern of respiratory bacterial pathogens isolated. *Haemophilus influenzae*, *Streptococcus pneumoniae* and *Moraxella catarrhalis* are usually implicated in patients with mild to moderate disease
- In patients admitted to hospital with community acquired pneumonia (CAP), assessment of initial pneumonia severity is important to guide decisions regarding site of care and initial empiric antibacterial treatment
- Patients with severe CAP should be treated with combination therapy, usually a broad spectrum β-lactam plus, either a macrolide or a respiratory quinolone antibiotic.

2.1 Introduction

Lower respiratory tract infections including community-acquired pneumonia (CAP) are very frequent in secondary care. For example,

, the incidence
...ched 7.7/1000
...ssions for acute
...uld be at least
...de, and adverse
...views key prin-
...tions.

...ions

...vith symptoms of
...spital may readily
...on testing and can
...e bronchitis, influ-
...onia. Chest radio-
...ing function testing

Patients with acute br..... ...aluated for influenza virus in the autumn/winter season for two reasons. First, the diagnosis of influenza may be relevant in terms of prevention of uncontrolled hospital spread. Second, patients presenting with an onset of symptoms of less than 36–48 hours may benefit from antiviral treatment with oseltamivir or zanamivir. Both agents shorten the length of symptoms by around 1 day.

Apart from influenza virus, acute bronchitis is usually caused by respiratory viruses such as rhinoviruses, respiratory syncytial viruses (RSV), parainfluenzaviruses, coronaviruses, human metapneumoviruses (HMPV), and adenoviruses. This is why antibacterial treatment is not indicated. Several placebo-controlled studies including penicillins, macrolides, and tetracyclines have shown no difference in outcome at the cost of excess toxicity. Unfortunately, these studies usually excluded elderly and more severely disabled patients. Therefore, in patients presenting with severe acute bronchitis and/or decompensated co-morbidity, a careful individual decision in favour of antibacterial treatment may be justified. Treatment is otherwise symptomatic, and may include antipyretics, antitussive agents, and fluid replacement.

2.2.3 Acute exacerbation of COPD

Patients with COPD frequently develop acute exacerbations, presenting mainly as a deterioration in general state, increase of cough, sputum volume, dyspnoea, and/or change of sputum colour. In the absence of distinctive quantitative criteria for an acute exacerbation, the diagnosis is made when the changes are severe enough to support a change in treatment.

All patients with acute exacerbations receive systemic steroids, either i.v. or orally, as well as nebulized short-acting bronchodilators. Aminophylline may be offered additionally. Depending on gas exchange as reflected by blood gasses, oxygen is indicated to correct hypoxaemia and ventilatory support to maintain ventilation.

Although considerable evidence has been provided in support of bacterial infection as the aetiology of acute exacerbations in around 50% of cases, and all authoritative guidelines recommend antibacterial treatment in patients with dyspnoea and purulent sputum, the benefit of this treatment is limited at best.

Recent data show that viral pathogens are present in the majority of patients with exacerbations, and bacterial pathogens found in respiratory secretions of around 50% of patients may represent pathogens as well as bystanders. The latter may origin from colonizing species present in up to 25% of patients with stable disease. However, a major step forward in the understanding of exacerbations has been the finding of the association of exacerbations with the acquisition of new bacterial strains. These newly acquired strains can only be detected by molecular techniques. As far as is known, around 20–25% of patients with exacerbations harbour a newly acquired pathogen.

On the other hand, placebo-controlled studies evaluating the effect of antibacterial agents show conflicting results. Whereas most do not demonstrate a benefit of antibacterial treatment, the landmark study by Anthonisen *et al.* suggests that there is a 20% benefit in terms of improvement of symptoms and airway obstruction compared to placebo for amoxicillin, tetracycline or co-trimoxazole in patients with severe COPD. Another study including patients with severe exacerbations treated at the ICU showed a survival benefit for antibacterial treatment with ofloxacin. However, that study is devalued by several major methodological flaws. Taken together, all available studies have major limitations which cannot be overcome by metanalyses. An alternative approach relying on the biomarker procalcitonin (PCT) demonstrated that a PCT-guided treatment reduced the number of patients needing antibacterial treatment to about 40%. This was the percentage of patients with some amount of inflammatory response as assessed by PCT. No information is available about the correlation of the inflammatory response with the presence of pathogens or even newly acquired pathogens.

The preliminary conclusion in view of these data should be to restrict antibacterial treatment to those patients with more severe acute exacerbations and/or COPD. Of note, a patient with severe COPD may experience a mild exacerbation and vice versa.

Whereas the severity of COPD is not always known at presentation of the patient, the severity of the acute exacerbation can be assessed. Unfortunately, there is currently no validated tool available for severity assessment. A reasonable albeit not systematically validated approach may be to rely on criteria including co-morbidity, performance status, need for oxygen supplementation, and need for ventilatory support. These simple criteria may allow judgements about the appropriate treatment setting (Table 2.1) and may also provide the basis for decisions about antibacterial treatment (Table 2.2). The indications for antibiotics according to this pathway are limited to patients with:

- Anthonisen type 1 and 2, mild exacerbations and severe COPD
- Anthonisen type 1 and 2, moderate exacerbations
- Severe exacerbations.

These indications closely follow the current available evidence in that most patients with mild exacerbations would not qualify for antibacterial treatment. Nevertheless, even these indications may be challenged by future tools to recognize those patients with newly acquired pathogens and a relevant inflammatory response.

Patients with an indication for antibacterial treatment should be treated along the expected microbial pattern. Recent data have confirmed an association between lung function and the pattern of pathogens isolated. *Haemophilus influenzae*, *Streptococcus pneumoniae* and *Moraxella catarrhalis* are usually implicated in patients with mild to moderate disease, whereas Gram-negative enterobacteriaceae (GNEB) and *Pseudomonas aeruginosa* are also implicated in patients with more advanced disease. Overall, resistant pathogens are more frequent in advanced disease as a result of previous antimicrobial treatment as well as hospitalizations.

Thus, patients with mild exacerbations should receive amoxicillin (or amoxicillin/β-lactamase inhibitor), macrolides, or tetracyclines. The available authoritative guidelines recommend empirical antipseudomonal treatment for patients with severe exacerbations. However, in contrast to pneumonia, patients with acute exacerbations are not at risk of severe sepsis and septic shock, and, therefore, do not run a risk of excess mortality in instances of inadequate initial empiric antibacterial treatment. Thus, our practice is to advocate amoxicillin/β-lactamase inhibitor (or a respiratory quinolone in situations of intolerance to β-lactams) as initial treatment in patients with severe exacerbations, carefully adapting treatment along the results of sputum cultures. There is some evidence supporting individual cycling of antibacterial agents in order to prevent the development of microbial resistance. This may be considered in patients with frequent acute exacerbations (3 or more per year).

Treatment duration should be strictly limited to 7 days. Patients with persisting instability after 7 days of treatment are in need of a diagnostic re-evaluation including repeated sputum cultures.

Table 2.1 Suggested severity assessment of acute exacerbation of COPD

Severity of exacerbation	Treatment setting	Comorbidity	Performance status	Need for oxygen supplementation	Need for ventilatory support
mild	ambulatory	stable	good	no	no
moderate	hospital	stable / unstable	intermediate / poor	yes*	no
severe	intermediate care / ICU	stable / unstable	intermediate / poor	yes*	yes**

* Patients on long-term oxygen treatment meet the criterion if the oxygen demand is increased.

** Patients on home ventilation meet the criterion if the ventilator settings must be changed or invasive ventilation is required.

Co-morbidity is a binary criterion only in the case of stable disease (supports mild exacerbation), performance only in the case of good performace (supports mild exacerbation).

Table 2.2 Indications for antibacterial treatment in acute exacerbations of COPD

Mild exacerbation			Moderate exacerbation		Severe exacerbation
Anthonisen 1+2		Anthonisen 3	Anthonisen 1+2	Anthonisen 3	antibiotic
COPD		no antibiotic	antibiotic	no antibiotic	
mild	moderate / severe				
no antibiotic	antibiotic				

Anthonisen 1 = increase in dyspnea, sputum volume, and change in sputum colour

Anthonisen 2 = two or three of these criteria

Anthonisen 3 = less than two of these criteria

In mild exacerbation, severity of COPD can be readily assessed by lung function testing.

2.3 Community-acquired pneumonia

2.3.1 Diagnosis

The diagnosis of community-acquired pneumonia (CAP) is usually straightforward since it requires symptoms of an acute respiratory infection together with a new infiltrate on chest radiography.

Recently, some authoritative statements have claimed that healthcare-associated pneumonia (HCAP) must be considered a new entity separate from CAP. The basic concept behind HCAP is that an increasing number of elderly and severely disabled patients experience pneumonia by multidrug-resistant (MDR) pathogens not covered in current recommendations of initial empiric antibacterial treatment, therefore resulting in excess mortality. However, the evidence for a link between increased mortality in these patients and inadequate initial empiric treatment due to MDR pathogens is weak, and certainly not substantiated in Europe.

Thus, it is still appropriate to address as CAP all immunocompetent patients with pneumonia acquired outside the hospital. Some caution is indicated in patients residing in nursing homes since a proportion of these patients may be at increased risk for meticillin-resistant *Staphylococcus aureus* (MRSA) and other multidrug-resistant (MDR) pathogens.

2.3.2 **Assessment of severity**

CAP carries a considerable risk of mortality, reaching 7–8% even in patients not residing in nursing homes and not bedridden. Mortality is twice in nursing home residents and thrice in bedridden patients. Therefore, it is important to assess initial pneumonia severity in order to guide decisions about treatment settings and initial empiric antibacterial treatment. Two tools for severity assessment have been proposed, the pneumonia severity index (PSI) by Fine *et al.* and the CURB-65 score and its modifications by Lim *et al.* Both operate similarly in classifying patients at risk of death. Since the CURB-65 is much easier to remember and to calculate, it is the preferable tool. A modification of the CURB-65 score, the CRB-65 score, allows the classification of the risk of mortality in a three class pattern, with mortality rates of 1–3% for CRB-65 class 1, 8–10% for class 2, and 30–35% for class 3. It is best applied as a tool to validate clinical judgment, and certainly, clinical judgment should always overrule any severity tool in cases of disparity.

The choice of treatment setting should widely follow the CRB-65 or CURB-65 scores. Thus, patients with CRB-65/ CURB-65 risk class 1 may safely be treated outside the hospital. There are, however, non-medical reasons to hospitalize patients, and a short period of hospitalization may be the right decision in cases of doubt. Patients with severe CAP are at a very high risk of death, reaching 30–40%. Again, several tools have been evaluated to predict patients with severe CAP. However, it has become evident that the decision to admit to the ICU is dependent on the local facilities and the resulting policies of ICU admission. Therefore, severity criteria are less useful to indicate the need for ICU admission but should be used to guide the extent of monitoring required, regardless whether this is applied in the ICU, in intermediate care units or even in general medical wards. The crucial indicators of severity include:

- Presence of acute respiratory failure (assessed by respiratory rate, blood gas analysis, or indices such as the PiO_2/FiO_2) with or without
- Presence of severe sepsis or septic shock (assessed by classical definitions according to Bone et al.).

Only patients requiring invasive ventilation and septic shock have an absolute indication for ICU admission unless there is an indication for treatment limitation due to severe and irreversible disability.

2.3.3 Diagnostic workup

Ambulatory patients do not need any additional diagnostic workup. They should, however, be reassessed at least 48 hours after initiation of antibacterial treatment. Hospitalized patients should receive oximetry or blood gas analysis, basic clinical chemistry including CRP or PCT, as well as blood cultures. Sputum cultures and antigen testing for *S. pneumoniae* and *Legionella pneumophila* serogroup 1 should be performed whenever possible. Bronchoscopy with bronchoalveolar lavage is usually restricted to mechanically ventilated patients.

2.3.4 Principles of antimicrobial treatment

Antimicrobial treatment is guided by pneumonia severity. This is not because severity determines pathogen patterns but because inadequate empiric treatment is associated with excess mortality in patients with severe pneumonia. Having said this, initial antimicrobial coverage will have to increase with increasing severity of pneumonia but also directed according to the results of microbiological investigations. This is called 'de-escalation strategy'.

Initial empiric antimicrobial treatment should always cover *S. pneumoniae* as the most frequent and potentially aggressive pathogen. *Haemophilus influenzae* as well as atypical pathogens such as *Legionella* sp, *Mycoplasma pneumoniae*, *Chlamydophila pneumoniae* and viruses have to be expected additionally. *Staphylococcus aureus* may be occasionally involved, particularly together with influenza virus. Gram-negative enterobacteriaceae (GNEB) and *P. aeruginosa* are exceedingly rare.

Treatment duration in cases of treatment response should be restricted to 7 days. The only exception is *Staph aureus* pneumonia with bacteremia and Legionellosis if treated with macrolides. Both of these conditions should be treated for at least 2 weeks. Although *P. aeruginosa* might recur, prolonged treatment has not been shown to decrease the risk of recurrence but increases the risk for development of resistance.

2.3.5 **Selection of initial empiric antimicrobial treatment**

In patients with mild pneumonia, regular coverage of atypical pathogens is probably not necessary. This is true even in the presence of *Legionella sp.* Therefore, oral amoxicillin/β-lactamase-inhibitor (or a respiratory quinolone in case of intolerance to β-lactams) are appropriate choices. Monotherapy with macrolides may be appropriate in younger patients without individual and regional risks for drug-resistant pneumococci.

Hospitalized patients without criteria for severe CAP should receive sequential (iv to oral) therapy. Initial intravenous treatment can be switched to oral treatment after 48–72 hours. A broad-spectrum β-lactam plus a macrolide or a respiratory quinolone are the principal choices. In cases of clinical response after 72 hours and where there is no evidence for *Legionella sp.*, consideration may be given to stopping the macrolide.

Patients with severe CAP should be treated with combination therapy, usually a broad-spectrum β-lactam plus a macrolide or plus a respiratory quinolone. De-escalation where appropriate should also be applied in these patients, and sequential therapy may be applied in patients without initial septic shock, in cases of clinical response and in the absence of malabsorption.

In patients at increased risk of *P. aeruginosa* (basically those with severe respiratory co-morbidity, repeated antimicrobial treatment and hospitalizations as well as severe disability including high risk of aspiration or enteral tube feeding), anti-pseudomonal combination therapy is indicated. Vancomycin should be considered as part of initial treatment in patients at risk for MRSA pneumonia (essentially patients with nasal carriage of MRSA). In these patients, it is particularly important to adhere to the principles of de-escalation in order to restrict selection pressure.

Treatment recommendations are listed in Table 2.3.

2.3.6 **Assessment of treatment response**

Treatment response is assessed at 48–72 hours. Criteria of stability in patients outside the ICU include: respiratory rate (<24/min), blood pressure (systolic pressure ≥90mmHg, diastolic pressure >60mmHg), heart rate (< 100/min), oxygenation (oxygen saturation ≥90%), and mental state (no confusion). The criteria of stability are at the same time the criteria for switch therapy. In addition, an assessment of inflammatory response by CRP or procalcitonin (PCT) may be performed; decreasing values indicate treatment response. All criteria should be met prior to hospital discharge. Full autonomy or, alternatively, home care should be ensured.

2.3.7 **Treatment failure**

In up to 10% of cases, treatment failure might occur. This may present as non-resolving pneumonia (persisting symptoms without

Table 2.3 Initial antimicrobial treatment in CAP			
Pneumonia severity	Treatment setting	Antibacterial treatment	Administration
mild	ambulatory	amoxicillin OR amoxicillin / β-lactamase-inhibitor OR moxifloxacin OR levofloxacin OR macrolide * (younger, no risk or resistance to S. pneumoniae)	orally
moderate	hospital	amoxicillin/ clavulanic acid or ceftriaxone ± macrolide * OR moxifloxacin levofloxacin	sequential treatment (i.v. / orally)
severe	hospital, monitored bed or ICU	ceftriaxone + macrolide * OR ceftriaxone + moxifloxacin or levofloxacin	sequential treatment (i.v. / orally)

Exceptionally, severe CAP with risk factors for *P. aeruginosa* will be empirically treated with: [piperacillin/tazobactam or carbapenem (imipenem or meropenem)] plus macrolide OR plus ciprofloxacin.
*erythromycin, clarithromycin or azithromycin

progression) or progressive pneumonia (clinical deterioration). Moreover, even despite initial treatment response, complications such as complicated parapneumonic effusion or empyema may emerge. The reasons behind treatment failure are complex and should prompt extensive expert re-evaluation.

Further reading

Bauer T.T., Ewig S., Marre R., Suttorp N., Welte T. (2006) The CAPNETZ Study Group. CRB-65 predicts death from community-acquired pneumonia. *J Intern Med* **260**: 93–101.

Blasi F., Ewig S., Torres A., Huchon G. (2006) A review of guidelines for anti-bacterial use in acute exacerbations of chronic bronchitis. *Pulm Pharmacol Ther* **19**: 361–9.

British Thoracic Society Standards of Care Committee. BTS Guidelines for the management of community acquired pneumonia in adults. *Thorax* **64**(3): 1–55.

Ewig S., Birkner N., Strauss R., *et al.* (2009) New perspectives on community-acquired pneumonia in 388,406 patients. *Thorax* **64**(12):1062–9.

Lim W.S., van der Eerden M.M., Laing R., *et al.* (2003) Defining community acquired pneumonia severity on presentation to hospital: an international derivation and validation study. *Thorax* **58**: 377–82.

Mandell L.A., Wunderink R.G., Anzueto A., *et al.* (2007) Infectious Diseases Society of America; American Thoracic Society. Infectious Diseases Society of America/American Thoracic Society consensus guidelines on the management of community-acquired pneumonia in adults. *Clin Infect Dis* **44**(2): S27–72.

Papi A., Bellettato C.M., Braccioni F., *et al.* (2006) Infections and airway inflammation in chronic obstructive pulmonary disease severe exacerbations. *Am J Respir Crit Care Med* **173**: 1114–21.

Sethi S., Sethi R., Eschberger K., *et al.* (2007) Airway bacterial concentrations and exacerbations of chronic obstructive pulmonary disease. *Am J Respir Crit Care Med* **176**: 356–61.

Sethi S., Wrona C., Eschberger K., Lobbins P., Cai X., Murphy T.F. (2008) Inflammatory profile of new bacterial strain exacerbations of chronic obstructive pulmonary disease. *Am J Respir Crit Care Med* **177**: 491–7.

Woodhead M., Blasi F., Ewig S., *et al.* (2005) European Respiratory Society; European Society of Clinical Microbiology and Infectious Diseases. Guidelines for the management of adult lower respiratory tract infections. *Eur Respir J* **26**: 1138–80.

Chapter 3

Hospital-acquired pneumonia

John Simpson

> **Key points**
> - Hospital-acquired pneumonia (HAP) is the most commonly fatal nosocomial infection
> - The diagnosis of HAP is difficult on clinical grounds but should be suspected when a patient develops infiltrates on a chest x-ray 2 days or more into hospital stay along with leukocytosis, pyrexia, or purulent respiratory secretions
> - Appropriate antibiotics should be given promptly when HAP is strongly suspected (with, if at all possible, an attempt to obtain lower respiratory tract secretions immediately beforehand)
> - The risk of antibiotic-resistant pathogens being responsible for HAP increases with length of stay in hospital, increased severity of illness, prior use of antibiotics, and recent contact with medical services
> - Several patient-specific and iatrogenic factors increase the risk of HAP, many of which can be modified to improve prevention.

3.1 Introduction

Hospital-acquired pneumonia (HAP) is an important condition that presents doctors with significant clinical challenges. This largely stems from difficulties inherent in making a confident diagnosis, the broad range of potentially responsible micro-organisms, and the relatively small evidence base informing decision-making. Most of the available literature is centred upon pneumonia in intubated patients requiring mechanical ventilation (ventilation-associated pneumonia (VAP)). Much less is known about the larger population of patients who develop HAP outside the intensive care unit (ICU). This chapter attempts to provide an overview of the epidemiology, microbiology, diagnosis, treatment, and prevention of HAP while highlighting key controversies. In recent years the terms healthcare-associated pneumonia (HCAP) and nursing home-acquired pneumonia (NHAP) have emerged in response to the fact that pneumonia acquired in specific settings outside hospital may behave differently from community-acquired pneumonia. HCAP and NHAP are not dealt with in this chapter.

3.2 Definitions

HAP is defined as pneumonia arising 48 hours or more into a hospital stay (effectively excluding the possibility that community-acquired infection was incubating at the time of admission).

VAP is defined as pneumonia arising 48 hours or more after mechanical ventilation. VAP is therefore a form of HAP (except in rare circumstances where ventilation is provided outside hospital).

3.3 Epidemiology

HAP is the second commonest nosocomial infection and is generally considered to arise in approximately 1% of hospital admissions. VAP may arise in up to 20% of intubated and mechanically ventilated patients.

HAP is associated with a higher crude mortality rate than any other nosocomial infection (typically around 30%). HAP (as opposed to the pre-existing illness) is thought to contribute up to 50% towards the observed mortality.

HAP is estimated to add approximately one week to hospital stay and is associated with considerable costs (typical estimates suggest that an episode of VAP costs in excess of $40,000 in the United States).

3.4 Pathogenesis and risk factors

During hospital admission, the oropharynx and nasopharynx are commonly colonized with potential respiratory pathogens. With increasing severity of illness and duration of hospital stay a higher frequency of antibiotic-resistant colonizing organisms are found. Colonizing micro-organisms may enter the lower respiratory tract by aspiration or through direct introduction (e.g. via an infected endotracheal tube). Aspiration often occurs repeatedly and in low volume (micro-aspiration) in patients who typically have impaired innate immune defences in the lung. The gastrointestinal tract may contribute significantly to aspiration of infected secretions and some authorities suggest a contribution from infected sinuses also.

HAP generally results in patchy bronchopneumonia which has important implications for the detection (or not) of pathogens using diagnostic sampling techniques, as discussed in Section 3.6.

Risk factors for HAP can broadly be divided into patient-specific and iatrogenic components (Table 3.1). Excessive use of antibiotics and (in the context of VAP) intubation are among the most consistently identified and important risk factors.

Table 3.1 Risk factors for HAP

Patient-specific	Iatrogenic
Smoking	Prior use of antibiotics
Lung disease	Intubation and mechanical ventilation
Renal insufficiency	Nasogastric tube
Diabetes mellitus	Surgery (especially thoracic and upper abdominal)
Shock	Sedation
Coma	Supine position
Malnutrition	Poor staff hand hygiene
Advancing age	Contaminated medical equipment (e.g. ventilator tubing)
Head trauma	
Male sex	Paralysing agents
Dental plaque	Enteral nutrition
	Red cell transfusions
	Treatments that raise gastric pH
	Moving ill patients between units

3.5 Microbiology

A wide range of micro-organisms are implicated in HAP (Table 3.2). Crucially, it is extremely difficult to generalize reports in the literature to your unit/hospital. Worse still, microbiological epidemiology is likely to differ from hospital to hospital in the same town, and even from unit to unit in the same hospital. For these reasons microbiological surveillance within units in which HAP is common is highly recommended in order to inform management decisions.

The majority of HAP is caused by bacteria and most series place Gram-negative pathogens as the main contributors. A variable but important proportion of HAP is polymicrobial. Whether anaerobes and fungi contribute to HAP is keenly debated, but their overall contribution seems to be small at most. The contribution of viruses to HAP has received insufficient attention for clear conclusions to be drawn.

Several studies have carefully assessed whether particular bacteria predominate in specific clinical settings (e.g. *Staphylococcus aureus* in patients with trauma), but it remains extremely difficult to predict the offending organism(s) on clinical grounds. Certain specific organisms have received particular attention in the literature. *Pseudomonas aeruginosa* is commonly implicated in HAP and associated with high rates of antibiotic resistance. *S. aureus* is also commonly implicated, and meticillin-resistant *S. aureus* (MRSA) presents particular implications for choice of treatment as discussed below. VAP in particular has been associated with increasingly virulent and antibiotic-resistant bacteria, such as *Acinetobacter baumannii*. The clinical importance and resistance patterns of major organisms significantly influences general recommendations for treatment of HAP. However it cannot be emphasized enough that good microbiological sampling in patients (where possible) and continuous high quality microbiological profiling within units are the most powerful tools in guiding therapy.

Table 3.2 Micro-organisms implicated in HAP
Gram-negative
*Escherichia coli**
*Haemophilus influenzae**
Klebsiella species*
Enterobacter species*
Proteus species*
*Serratia marcescens**
Moraxella species*
Pseudomonas aeruginosa
Acinetobacter species
Legionella species
Stenotrophomonas maltophilia
Neisseria species
Gram-positive
*Streptococcus pneumoniae**
Streptococcus species*
Meticillin-sensitive *Staphylococcus aureus**
Coagulase-negative Staphylococci*
Meticillin-resistant *Staphylococcus aureus*
Other
Anaerobes
Fungi
Viruses
* denotes bacteria commonly isolated in 'early-onset' HAP, occurring within 5 days of hospital admission

3.6 Diagnosis

The diagnosis of HAP is notoriously difficult. No pathognomonic features exist and a wide variety of inflammatory pulmonary conditions can mimic HAP. The fundamental problem is that HAP is infection of the gas-exchanging regions of the lung and this is very hard to confirm in patients. Strictly speaking histology is the 'gold standard' for pneumonia, and positive culture of pneumonic tissue confirms an infective pneumonia—clearly this is impractically invasive for all but a tiny minority of patients. The clinician is left with the dilemma of deciding how much clinical information is required to yield sufficient confidence that infective pneumonia is present (and if so which organism(s) is/are likely to be responsible).

HAP is suspected clinically if a patient has:

• New alveolar infiltrates on chest x-ray (CXR, see Figure 3.1) and one or more of the following:

• Temperature >38°C (or <36°C)

• Leukoctyosis (or leukopenia)

• Purulent lower respiratory tract secretions.

Particularly in VAP it is important to stipulate that the CXR infiltrates should be persistent (in order to exclude pulmonary oedema as the cause). Studies have suggested that in the presence of alveolar infiltrates on CXR and all three of the other conditions above, the accuracy of the clinical diagnosis of VAP is relatively high. Even with this heightened confidence however, the clinician is still faced with the question of which organism is responsible. This in turn leads to the vexed question of whether and how to obtain samples for microbiological analysis.

Sampling options can be broadly divided into an 'invasive' bronchoscopic approach (directed bronchoalveolar lavage (BAL) or protected specimen brush (PSB)) or a reasonably non-invasive approach (endotracheal aspirate (ETA) or sputum production (whether voluntary or induced by nebulizing hypertonic saline)). Invasive techniques sample the gas-exchanging regions of the lung much more reliably but are potentially dangerous (in already sick patients), dependent on skilled operators being available, and time consuming (so potentially delaying treatment). Non-invasive techniques, particularly ETA, generate samples of questionable relevance—i.e. is it reasonable to make inferences about the alveolar regions of the lung from a sample collected from the trachea? ETA is certainly responsible for a high rate of false positive 'infections' with the consequent risk of prescribing unnecessary antibiotics. The 'invasive versus non-invasive' debate is unresolved but has been informed by randomized controlled trials (RCTs). An impressive RCT conducted in French ICUs demonstrated both lower antibiotic prescribing and improved 14-day mortality in VAP using an invasive strategy, but this finding has not been consistently reproduced and most guidelines do not recommend routine use of an invasive approach.

In many respects the invasive versus non-invasive debate depends on pragmatism. Outside the ICU on hospital wards (where most HAP occurs) it is almost always impractical to arrange bronchoscopic tests.

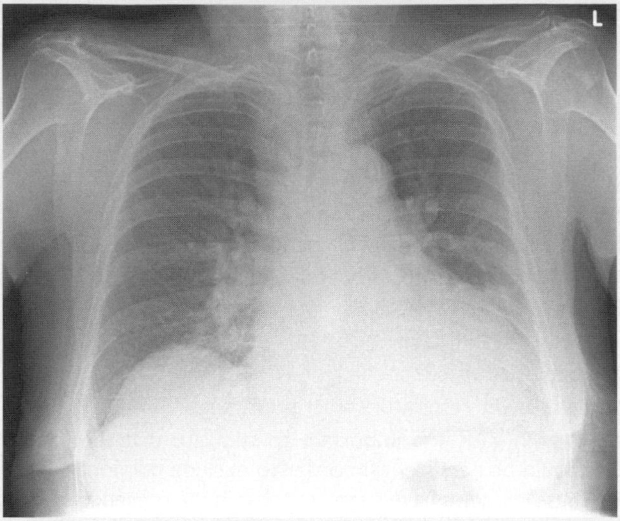

(a)

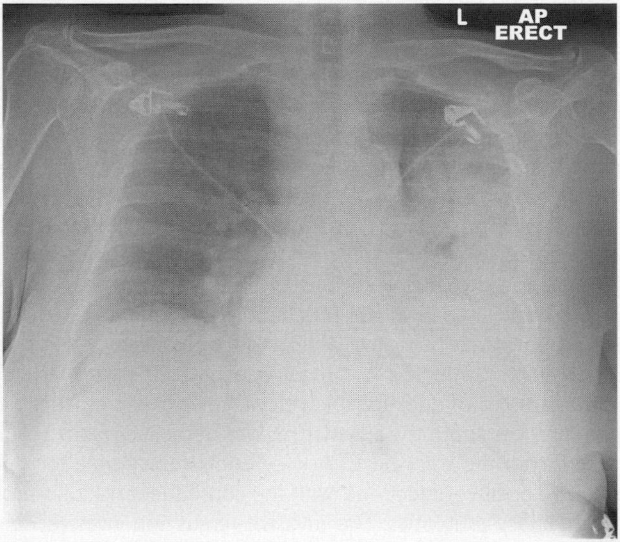

(b)

Figure 3.1 Radiological changes consistent with HAP. An elderly lady who had been in hospital for a week became breathless, developed a fever, and had increasing oxygen requirements. Her admission CXR is shown above, and the CXR taken a week later is shown below. The second CXR shows left-sided consolidation with air bronchograms and obscuring of the heart border, consistent with HAP. Courtesy of Dr J Murchison, Consultant Radiologist, Royal Infirmary of Edinburgh.

The issue then is whether to obtain samples at all, or to treat the patient empirically with the high attendant risk of unnecessary prescribing of antibiotics and the consequent effect on antibiotic resistance. Most authorities recommend a rapid attempt at obtaining a non-invasive sample without delaying empirical treatment, as discussed again below. However in most patients no adequate sample will be obtained.

The situation in ICUs is different as bronchoscopy is more readily available. Given the issues of time, operator availability and safety, techniques such as 'non-bronchoscopic lavage' are emerging where a thin catheter is introduced blindly and a non-directed 'mini-BAL' performed. These simpler methods of alveolar sampling need to be rigorously compared with directed, bronchoscopic techniques and non-invasive techniques. Ultimately however, all sampling techniques are restrained by lack of understanding of what is going on at the alveolar level. HAP is not only a patchy process but a dynamic and rapidly changing one, in which bacterial populations vary over time and the host inflammatory response may have an important bearing on outcome. Under these circumstances better imaging to guide sampling might help (but is again often impractical). However the great hope remains the identification of biomarkers, preferably in blood, which are specific for pneumonia. The search continues with some promising candidates emerging.

In the meantime, the general advice is to obtain good quality microbiological samples whenever possible in suspected HAP, but not to allow this to delay treatment. Samples should be sent fresh to a microbiology laboratory experienced in nosocomial pathogens and performing quantitative cultures. Quantitative culture improves specificity for the diagnosis of HAP (i.e. relevant pathogens at $>10^4$ colony forming units (CFU) per ml of BAL fluid, $>10^3$ CFU/ml of PSB fluid, and even $>10^6$ CFU/ml of ETA greatly increase diagnostic confidence for VAP).

3.7 **Treatment**

When HAP is suspected on clinical and radiographic grounds, the principles of treatment are to obtain a microbiological sample immediately if possible, initiate antibiotics promptly, and observe the patient's response carefully. The clinician must simultaneously weigh up multiple patient-specific factors. It is well recognized that the risk of antibiotic-resistant pathogens is higher if the patient is severely ill or has been in hospital for five days or more. Other risk factors for the presence of multidrug-resistant pathogens have been described, for example prescription of antibiotics in the previous three months or recent contact with medical services. Finally, and crucially, the clinician should be aware of the microbiological epidemiology of the unit/hospital and must communicate with local microbiologists to obtain results from submitted samples.

These principles have informed recent guidelines which are broadly similar in their approach. In general these guidelines advocate stratification based on the risk of multidrug resistance. Welcome trends include a move towards monotherapy and for courses of antibiotics to last no longer than 8 days, except in instances where the risk of multidrug resistance is felt to be exceptionally high (e.g. when there is an appreciably high rate of MRSA in the unit). An example algorithm for the treatment of HAP is shown in Figure 3.2. UK guidelines have recommended a slightly less aggressive approach and would advocate co-amoxiclav or cefuroxime for Group 1 in Figure 3.1, with less emphasis on carbapenems for Group 2.

As described in Section 3.6, high quality microbiological samples will usually be unavailable. Existing guidelines readily accept that empirical therapy without sampling will lead to many patients getting unnecessary antibiotics (and by implication the inflammatory condition mimicking HAP will remain untreated). Recent data have suggested that empirical, guideline-based treatment in the ICU may even potentially have an adverse effect on outcomes. For these reasons patients must be monitored closely in the first 72 hours of treatment with a view to withdrawing empirical antibiotics where possible. In particular some centres use a 12-point clinical pulmonary infection score (CPIS) to direct empirical therapy, such that antibiotics are withdrawn if the CPIS is less than 6 at baseline and again at 72 hours (see Further Reading for details). Similarly guidelines recommend rationalization of antibiotics according to returning microbiological results.

3.8 **Prevention**

Prevention follows the principles of ensuring cleanliness and avoiding aspiration (or direct introduction of bacteria) into the respiratory tract. Handwashing, the use of gloves, institutional infection control programmes, and preventive 'bundles' can all have positive effects.

Avoidance of intubation and nasogastric tubes wherever possible is a key objective. Semi-recumbent positioning of patients at 30°–45° reduces the risk of aspiration. A variety of ventilation-specific measures may reduce the incidence of VAP (e.g. subglottic drainage, infrequent changes of ventilator tubing etc).

Decontamination of the mouth using chlorhexidine appears to be of benefit in selected patients (e.g. after cardiac surgery). Wherever possible stress ulcer prophylaxis (e.g. with antacids) should be avoided as these raise gastric pH promoting overgrowth of bacteria and a potential infective source of aspiration. More controversial is the practice of using oral (with or without systemic) antibiotics to achieve 'selective digestive decontamination'. Most guidelines discourage the routine use of this practice.

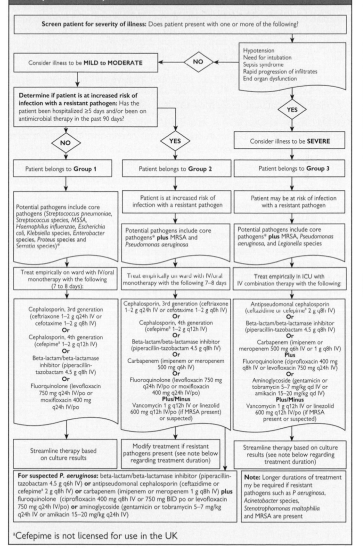

Figure 3.2 Treatment algorithm for hospital-acquired pneumonia (Reproduced from C Rotstein, G Evans, A Born, et al. Clinical practice guidelines for hospital aquired pneumonia and ventilator associated pneumonia in adults. *The Canadian Journal of Infectious Diseases and Medical Microbiology,* January/February 2008, Volume 19 Issue 1: 19–53. © Pulsus Group Inc., 2008).

Further reading

American Thoracic Society/Infectious Disease Society of America (2005) Guidelines for the management of adults with hospital-acquired, ventilator-associated, and healthcare-associated pneumonia. *Am J Respir Crit Care Med* **171**: 388–416.

Anand N. Kollef M.H. (2009) The alphabet soup of pneumonia: CAP, HAP, HCAP, NHAP, and VAP. *Semin Respir Crit Care* **30**: 3–9.

Canadian Critical Trials Group (2006) A randomized trial of diagnostic techniques for ventilator-associated pneumonia. *N Engl J Med* **355**: 2619–30.

Chastre J., Fagon J.Y. (2002) Ventilator-associated pneumonia. *Am J Respir Crit Care Med* **165**: 867–903.

Fagon J.Y., Chastre J., Wolff M., *et al.* (2000) Invasive and noninvasive strategies for management of suspected ventilator-associated pneumonia A randomized trial. *Ann Intern Med* **132**: 621–30.

Kett D.H., Cano E., Quartin A.A. *et al.* (2011) Implementation of guidelines for management of possible multi-drug resistant pneumonia in intensive care: an observational, multicentre cohort study. *Lancet Infect Dis* **11**: 181–89.

Masterton R.G. Galloway A. French G., *et al.* (2008) Guidelines for the management of hospital-acquired pneumonia in the UK. *J Antimicrob Chemother* **62**: 5–34.

Rotstein C. Evans G., Born A., *et al.* (2008) Clinical practice guidelines for hospital-acquired pneumonia and ventilator-associated pneumonia in adults. *Can J Infect Dis Med Microbiol* **19**: 19–53.

Singh N., Rogers P., Atwood C.W., Wagener M.M., Yu V.L. (2000) Short-course antibiotic therapy for patients with pulmonary infiltrates in the intensive care unit. A proposed solution for indiscriminate antibiotic prescription. *Am J Respir Crit Care Med* **162**(2Pt1): 505–11.

Chapter 4

The immunocompromised host: (a) patients with HIV

Morgan Evans and Pradhib Venkatesan

> **Key points**
> - Respiratory infections are common in HIV patients
> - Respiratory presentations are an opportunity to diagnose HIV infection for the first time
> - *Pneumocystis jirovecii* infection differs from bacterial pneumonia in having a subacute onset
> - Tuberculosis and HIV co-infection affects 1.1 million people worldwide and is a major cause of morbidity and mortality
> - Bacterial pneumonia from *Streptococcus pneumoniae* is commoner in HIV patients than some opportunistic pathogens.

4.1 Introduction

Highly active anti-retroviral treatment has made a dramatic difference to the lives of patients infected with human immunodeficiency virus (HIV). Patients well controlled on treatment are not experiencing opportunistic infections and are living longer lives. Respiratory presentations may reflect their longer life span and include lung cancer or heart failure following a myocardial infarct. Patients with HIV have an increased incidence of particular cancers and cardiovascular events. However for some patients the diagnosis of HIV and the commencement of anti-retroviral therapy occur after presentation with an opportunistic infection. Respiratory infections are common causes of such presentations. Some respiratory pathogens only present when there is significant immunocompromise, e.g. *Pneumocystis jirovecii*. Other pathogens may present with either reduced or normal immunity, e.g. *Mycobacterium tuberculosis*.

4.2 **Clinical presentation**

4.2.1 **Diagnosing HIV**

In a patient known to be HIV positive the range of pathogens, respiratory syndromes, and the clinical approach are well defined. When a patient with undiagnosed HIV presents with a respiratory infection there is the challenge of recognizing the possibility of HIV and immunocompromise. Delays in making the right diagnosis and instituting the right treatment can cost lives. In the past the possibility of HIV was prompted when patients were in a 'risk group', e.g. men who have sex with men (MSM) and intravenous drug users (IVDUs). Increasingly HIV has become a heterosexual epidemic and in some countries key heterosexual groups are immigrants from high endemicity countries. Prompts to think about immunocompromise and HIV infection may come from oral thrush, oral hairy leukoplakia, persistent lymphadenopathy, herpes zoster infection at a young age, diarrhoea and weight loss, recurrent infections, persistent skin problems, and a raised ESR at a young age. In a UK and Ireland questionnaire survey Sullivan *et al.* (2005) found that a clue was present in 17% of patients over the 12 months prior to their HIV diagnosis.

The prompt to think about immunocompromise and HIV may come from finding a pathogen only associated with immunocompromise, e.g. *P. jirovecii*. Other pathogens are being added to the list of indicators for an HIV test. Some national guidelines state that tuberculosis is an indication for an HIV test and that this should also be considered for bacterial pneumonia and aspergillosis.

4.2.2 **Clinical syndromes**

For any hospitalized respiratory illness a chest X ray (CXR) is performed. Different patterns of CXR changes are seen. Table 4.1 lists a range of pathogens seen in HIV patients and the possible CXR patterns they may cause. As with any such table the listings are not definitive but suggestive. For some infections a very poor immune response may not produce the inflammatory change required for CXR shadowing. Both *P. jirovecii* and *M. tuberculosis* have been associated with infection but entirely clear CXRs.

Certain clinical features may be suggestive of the cause. Bacterial pneumonias usually progress over a few days and a short history is typical. Atypical pathogens may present gradually but the history is still less than 10–14 days. However in HIV, opportunistic pathogens often progress more gradually with illness lasting longer than 2 weeks. This is found with *M. tuberculosis* and *P. jirovecii*. The probability of the latter two pathogens is affected by exposure history and prophylaxis. Tuberculosis is mainly seen in patients with exposure in an area of high endemicity. Good adherence to co-trimoxazole *Pneumocystis* prophylaxis renders this a less likely infection with CD4 counts less than 200 cells/mm³. The CD4 count measures the T lymphocyte subset mainly affected by HIV. The virus targets CD4 + cells and depletes their numbers. Patients with CD4 counts <200 cells/mm³ are particularly vulnerable to a wide range of pathogens.

Table 4.1 Respiratory pathogens and CXR patterns seen in HIV patients

Pathogen	Diffuse interstitial infiltrates	Focal consolidation	Cavities	Nodules or masses	Lymphadenopathy	Pleural effusion
Viruses						
CMV	+					
Influenza	+					
Bacteria						
S. pneumoniae		+				+
H. influenzae		+				
Legionella		+				
Pseudomonas		+	+			
St. aureus		+	+			+
Rhodococcus		+	+			
Nocardia		+		+		
M. tuberculosis	+	+	+	+	+	+
Atypical mycobacteria		+				
Fungi						
P. jirovecii	+		+			
Cryptococcus	+		+	+		
Aspergillus		+	+	+		
Histoplasma	+	+	+	+	+	+
Penicillium		+	+			
Coccidioides	+				+	
Protozoa						
Toxoplasma	+					

4.2.3 Investigation

Given the variety of pathogens, investigation to elucidate the cause and institute the right treatment is important. In addition to routine blood tests and cultures it may be important to obtain a deep respiratory sample for microbiology by induced sputum or from bronchoscopy. CT scans may define patterns and lesions to target for biopsy. The pathogen may not be confined to the chest and seeking specimens elsewhere can be helpful.

4.3 *Pneumocystis jirovecii*

P. jirovecii is an environmental fungus commonly inhaled but only the cause of disease in the immunocompromised. It is usually seen when the CD4 count is <200 cells/mm^3. It remains a common reason for hospitalization.

The onset of illness is usually subacute with malaise, fatigue, progressive shortness of breath, a non-productive cough, and low grade fever developing over a few weeks. Chest auscultation may be completely normal. Diffuse interstitial disease results in hypoxaemia and patients may be tachypnoeic. On exercise they desaturate quickly. Lung destruction may lead to cyst formation. Sudden shortness of breath and chest pain may indicate rupture of a cyst and a pneumothorax. CXR typically shows a bilateral perihilar interstitial infiltrate which progresses outwards to give a 'bats wing' appearance. Sometimes CXR changes are subtle (Figure 4.1). Pleural effusions and lymphadenopathy are rare.

P. jirovecii is not cultured and the diagnosis is usually dependent on visualizing the organism on staining or immunofluorescence. The organism disintegrates in expectorated sputum and deep samples are required. These may be obtained through sputum induction using a 3% hypertonic saline nebulizer and the help of a physiotherapist. The diagnostic yield is 50–90%. Alternatively bronchoscopy with bronchoalveolar lavage can provide a yield of > 95%. Transbronchial biopsy is not routinely performed because of the risk of pneumothorax. Some centres routinely use polymerase chain reaction (PCR) on respiratory samples instead of microscopy, but this sensitive test may be positive in the absence of *P. jirovecii* disease. PCR on serum samples is the subject of investigation. Some patients are too sick to tolerate respiratory sampling and serum based diagnosis would be beneficial.

The treatment of pneumocystis pneumonia is usually commenced before confirmation, based on the clinical picture. First line therapy is co-trimoxazole (commencing at 120 mg/kg/day in 3–4 divided doses) which may be used orally or intravenously depending on severity. Other options are clindamycin 600 mg qds plus primaquine (unlicensed in UK) 15–30 mg od, pentamidine 3–4 mg/kg/day or atovaquone 750mg bd. Clinical response may not be apparent for one week. If there is a failure to respond after one week one could switch from co-trimoxazole to another regime. Whether to do so is debateable. Co-trimoxazole is probably the most active drug and one may have to exercise patience. However a clear indication for

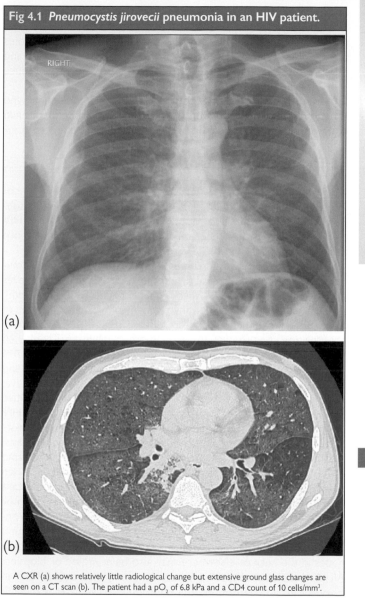

Fig 4.1 *Pneumocystis jirovecii* pneumonia in an HIV patient.

(a)

(b)

A CXR (a) shows relatively little radiological change but extensive ground glass changes are seen on a CT scan (b). The patient had a pO$_2$ of 6.8 kPa and a CD4 count of 10 cells/mm^3.

change is the occurrence of a drug reaction. This occurs regularly with co-trimoxazole, usually in the second week of treatment.

When *P. jirovecii* killing commences following treatment, there is an increase in lung inflammation. Consequently, an already hypoxaemic patient may be tipped into respiratory failure. To dampen the inflammatory response, high-dose steroids are indicated simultaneously with anti-fungal treatment when the pO_2 is <9.3 kPa. Steroids are typically commenced at a dose of prednisolone 40 mg bd and tapered to zero over 21 days. They have been shown to reduce mortality and the need for ventilation.

Mortality from pneumocystis pneumonia is 10–20%. Patients who deteriorate and require ventilation can still survive, with one US study quoting a hospital survival rate of 40% for such patients.

4.4 **Mycobacterium tuberculosis**

Worldwide in 2009 an estimated 1.1 million people were co-infected with both HIV and TB, with 80% of these living in sub-Saharan Africa. In that year about 380,000 people died from HIV associated TB. In the presence of HIV, active TB is 20–30 times more likely to develop than in those who are HIV negative.

The presentation of tuberculosis in patients with reduced immunity is less often the classical syndrome of prolonged cough, fever and weight loss, particularly when the CD4 count is <200 cells/mm^3. Appearances on CXR include involvement of a greater number of lobes, pleural effusions and miliary disease (Figure 4.2). Laboratory confirmation using sputum smears is more problematic. There is an increase in the proportion of patients whose smears are negative by traditional Ziehl-Neelsen (ZN) staining. Auramine staining and fluorescent techniques can be better. Historically, smear negative, HIV negative patients had a less severe course than smear positive patients, reflecting their lower mycobacterial burden. However, HIV positive patients with smear negative tuberculosis have a higher mortality, especially in resource poor countries, due to delayed diagnosis.

This makes the use of culture even more important, and rapid liquid culture techniques have been of great benefit in resource rich countries. When patients are unable to expectorate it is important to obtain a sample for culture and sensitivity. Sputum induction or bronchoscopy and bronchoalveolar lavage are useful. Prior to bronchoscopy a CT scan of the thorax may be performed to define a lymph node or other lesion which may be biopsied. Palpable lymph nodes in the neck or elsewhere may also be aspirated or biopsied. All of these sophisticated investigations may not be available in resource poor countries and this contributes to worldwide mortality from tuberculosis. The World Health Organization is investing in the use of PCR based diagnosis, with new techniques for rapidly diagnosing smear negative patients and drug resistant isolates.

The treatment of HIV associated tuberculosis remains broadly similar to non-HIV patients. There are a few caveats. In the UK *M. tuberculosis* drug resistance rates are slightly higher in HIV positive patients. Rapid detection of rifampicin resistance through molecular

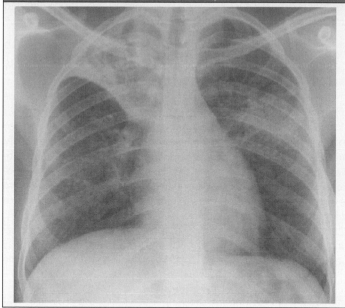

Fig 4.2 **A CXR of a patient with smear positive tuberculosis and HIV. This patient had a good CD4 count of 847 cells/mm³. Appearances are similar to a non-HIV patient**

probes is important. Patients with HIV are more prone to drug side effects. Skin rash and liver function test disturbance occur regularly. Patients with HIV may also be co-infected with hepatitis B or C and the liver toxicity of tuberculosis drugs can be problematic. Peripheral neuropathy occurs with HIV infection itself or with some anti-retrovirals. It is imperative that HIV patients on isoniazid are given pyridoxine routinely. With these caveats, standard tuberculosis treatment regimes are used as with non-HIV patients.

An added issue is drug interactions between tuberculosis treatment (rifampicin in particular) and anti-retroviral drugs (protease inhibitors in particular). These interactions require adjustments of dose or avoidance of some combinations of drugs. For new HIV diagnoses the initiation of anti-retrovirals can cause problems. Restoring CD4 cell function and numbers enhances the inflammatory response. This can result in an immune reconstitution inflammatory syndrome (IRIS). With tuberculosis, suppuration of lymph nodes, new pulmonary infiltrates and new pleural effusions have been described. Provided other causes have been excluded steroids have been used to reduce inflammation.

In smear positive HIV subjects a distinction must be made between *M. tuberculosis* and atypical mycobacteria. Molecular probes for the

M. tuberculosis complex can make this distinction and these are more readily used in HIV patients. *Mycobacterium avium* complex causes a systemic febrile illness and diagnosis may be made from mycobacterial blood cultures. Other atypical mycobacteria may be confined to the lung such as *Mycobacterium kansasii* and *Mycobacterium simiae*.

4.5 **Bacterial pneumonia**

In studies of respiratory infection in HIV, bacterial pneumonia and bronchitis are the commonest. Infections with *Streptococcus pneumoniae* (Figure 4.3) and *Haemophilus influenzae* are about 50 times commoner than in non-HIV controls. CD4 positive T cells are not directly involved in defence against these bacteria. However, during the course of HIV infection there can be disturbance of B lymphocyte function and antibody production. This does not parallel CD4 cell counts and pneumococcal infection can occur at any CD4 count. In late stage HIV there is also disturbance of neutrophil function. The latter predisposes to infection with *Pseudomonas sp.*

Invasive pneumococcal disease with bacteraemia is commoner in HIV and is associated with increased mortality. Protection may be provided through pneumococcal vaccination although in vaccine

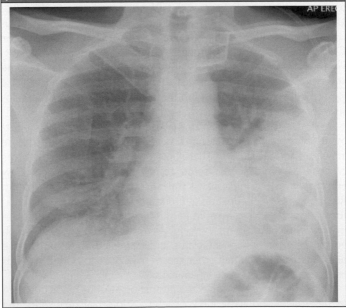

Fig 4.3 **A CXR** of pneumococcal pneumonia in a patient with HIV. *Streptococcus pneumoniae* was cultured from blood. The patient had a **CD4 count of 238 cells / mm³**

trials with HIV patients, the clinical efficacy has varied from benefit to detriment. Vaccine response depends on CD4 count and those with counts >200 cells/mm^3 are likely to benefit.

Infection with *S. pneumoniae* or *H. influenzae* is treated with standard antibiotics but some bacteria require combinations of drugs and prolonged treatment. These include *Nocardia sp.* and *Rhodococcus equi*. Both are commoner in HIV infection. Initial clinical features with the latter pathogens may be suggestive of tuberculosis.

4.6 **Fungal infections**

Some fungal infections are ubiquitous and others are endemic to certain localities. *P. jirovecii*, *Cryptococcus neoformans* and *Aspergillus sp.* are ubiquitous. *Cryptococcus* is inhaled from the environment, passes through the lung, and usually presents with meningitis. However respiratory infection may occur. *Aspergillus sp.* are seen in the very immunocompromised causing progressive and invasive infection of airways and the lung (see Section 5.9.1).

Fungal infections endemic in certain areas include *Coccidioides immitis* from the Americas, *Penicillium marneffei* from South East Asia, and *Histoplasma capsulatum* from regions outside Europe. *Coccidioides* and *Histoplasma* can cause a granulomatous inflammatory response and the clinical picture can overlap with tuberculosis.

4.7 **Viral infection**

Cytomegalovirus is more often a bystander in the lung in HIV than a key pathogen. It generally causes more problems in patients with other forms of immunosuppression, e.g. transplant recipients (see Section 5.9.4). However when found on tissue biopsy or by PCR, treatment is occasionally indicated.

Further reading

Briel M., Bucher H.C., Boscacci R., Furrer H. (2006) Adjunctive corticosteroids for *Pneumocystis jirovecii* pneumonia in patients with HIV-infection. *Cochrane Database of Systematic Reviews*, Issue 3.

British HIV Association and British Infection Association Guidelines for the Treatment of Opportunistic Infection in HIV-seropositive Individuals 2011. (2011) *HIV Medicine* **12**, (Suppl 2).

Centers for Disease Control and Prevention. (2009) Guidelines for Prevention and Treatment of Opportunistic Infections in HIV-Infected Adults and Adolescents. *Morbidity and Mortality Weekly Report* **58**, 1–216.

Curtis J.R., Yarnold P.R., Schwartz D.N., Weinstein R.A., Bennett C.L. (2000) Improvements in outcomes of acute respiratory failure for patients with Human Immunodeficiency Virus-related Pneumocystis carinii pneumonia. *Am J Respir Crit Care Med* **162**: 393–8.

Havlir D.V., Barnes P.F. (1999) Tuberculosis in patients with human immuno-deficiency virus infection. *N Engl J Med* **340**: 367–73.

Hull M.W., Phillips P., Montaner J.S. (2008) Changing global epidemiology of pulmonary manifestations of HIV/AIDS. *Chest* **134**: 1287–98.

Sullivan A.K., Curtis H., Sabin C.A., Johnson M.A. (2005) Newly diagnosed HIV infections: review in UK and Ireland. *Brit Med J* **330**: 1301–2.

Thomas C.F., Limper A.H. (2004) Pneumocystis pneumonia. *N Engl J Med* **350**: 2487–98.

UK National Guidelines for HIV Testing 2008. http://www.bhiva.org/files/file1031097.pdf.

Chapter 5

The immunocompromised host: (b) patients with haematological disorders

Jeremy Brown and James Brown

Key points

- Patients with haematological malignancy or who have had haematopoietic stem cell transplantation (HSCT) are often severely immunosuppressed, both due to the disease and as a result of the treatment
- Infectious complications affecting the respiratory tract are common and frequently severe in these patients
- There is a large range of pathogens that cause respiratory infections in haematology patients, and opportunistic infection with cytomegalovirus, *Aspergillus* species, and *Pneumocystis jirovecii* are common
- The likely microbial pathogen(s) can be narrowed down by assessment of the patient's underlying immune defect(s), the clinical presentation, the radiological features on the CT scan, and carefully targeted investigations
- Early use of empirical broad-spectrum antibiotics is essential in these patients if they present with symptoms or signs of a respiratory infection
- Expert advice is necessary unless there is a rapid response to empirical antibiotics.

5.1 Overview

Haematological malignancies and aplastic anaemia often cause severe immunosuppression, and this is compounded by their treatment which relies on intensive chemotherapy regimens or total marrow ablation followed by autologous or allograft HSCT. The newer biological therapies are also associated with very specific immune defects, e.g. B cell depletion after treatment with anti-CD20 monoclonal antibody. Hence patients with aplastic anaemia, undergoing HSCT (especially allografts), or receiving treatment for acute leukaemia or lymphoma frequently have prolonged defects in immunity. Patients with chronic leukaemia or multiple myeloma are also immunosuppressed, albeit usually to a lesser extent.

Furthermore, the effects of cytotoxic agents on respiratory epithelium integrity, replacement of the oropharyngeal microbial fauna with pathogenic organisms, and increased microaspiration in these patients all increase the risk of respiratory infection. Up to 60% of these patients will develop respiratory infections, which cause 5% of deaths post-HSCT. Immunosuppression not only increases the risk of infection but also markedly extends the range of potential pathogens that can cause respiratory infections. Relatively benign pathogens in the immunocompetent can cause severe disease in the immunosuppressed, making empirical therapy considerably more difficult.

This chapter provides a framework for managing haematology patients (and other non-HIV patients with severe immunosuppression) with respiratory infection. Whilst infections are common causes of pulmonary infiltrates in the immunocompromised, a range of non-infective causes also need to be considered, including:

- Pulmonary oedema
- Drug reactions
- Lung involvement by the underlying disease
- Aspiration
- Post-HSCT patients: diffuse alveolar haemorrhage, idiopathic pneumonia syndrome, lymphoproliferative disease, and engraftment syndrome.

5.2 **Clinical approach**

The organisms causing pulmonary infections in the severely immunocompromised host are listed in Box 5.1.

Although this large range of organisms is daunting, a systematic approach often identifies the likely pathogen(s) and most appropriate investigations, allowing targeted empirical therapy. This approach involves answering the following questions:

1. What type of immune defect(s) are present and their duration?
2. What are the salient clinical features, especially speed of onset?
3. What is the pattern of the lung infiltrate (best shown by a CT scan)?
4. Are there any other important factors (e.g. CMV status)?

Box 5.1 Pathogens associated with respiratory infections in haematology (and other severely immunosuppressed) patients

Viruses:	**16%**
CMV	6%
Respiratory viruses (parainfluenza, RSV, influenza, adenovirus, metapneumovirus)	8%
Bacteria:	**46%**
Gram negative (coliforms, *Pseudomonas*, other)	20%
Gram positive (*S. aureus*, streptococci species)	20%
Nocardia and mycobacteria	6%
Fungi:	**38%**
Pneumocystis jirovecii (PCP)	3%
Aspergillus species, other molds	26%
Candida species	9%
(adapted from Rañó et al. (2001) *Thorax* **56**:379–87)	

5.3 **Type of immune defect**

Recognition of the likely pathogen is essential to aid diagnosis and the correct choice of empirical therapy, and in the immunocompromised the likely pathogen is indicated by the patient's immune defect(s). These can be divided into defects affecting (a) neutrophils, (b) cell mediated immunity, or (c) antibody-dependent immunity. Immune defects can be caused by both treatment and the underlying disease, and patients may have a combination of defects that change over time. For instance, a patient with lymphoma may have background defects in cell mediated and antibody immunity due to the disease and then develop severe neutropenia after chemotherapy.

5.3.1 **Neutrophil defects**

Neutrophil defects (usually neutropenia) results in an increased susceptibility to:
- Gram negative and Gram positive extracellular bacteria
- Invasive aspergillosis and the rarer molds (e.g. *Mucor*, *Fusarium*), with the risk increasing with increasing duration of neutropenia
- Candidaemia with metastatic spread to the lungs

Causes of neutropenia include:
- Chemotherapy
- HSCT (early period, e.g. up to 2 weeks post-autologous and 4 weeks post-allograft)
- Disordered haemopoesis (acute myeloblastic leukaemia, chronic myelocytic anaemia, marrow infiltrations, aplastic anaemia).

In addition, functional defects of neutrophils can occur, either inherited (e.g. chronic granulomatous disease), or due to treatment with certain immunosupressives (azathioprine, mycophenolate, or high dose corticosteroids).

5.3.2 **Cell mediated immunity**

Defective or deficient T-cell mediated immunity causes increased susceptibility to intracellular and some opportunistic pathogens including:

- Viruses, mainly CMV and respiratory viruses
- Mycobacteria and *Nocardia*
- PCP
- Rarities, e.g. toxoplasmosis, endemic fungi (e.g. *Histoplasma*).

Causes of cell-mediated defects include:

- HSCT (prolonged period)
- Immunosuppressive drugs, e.g. tacrolimus, ciclosporin, azathioprine, high-dose corticosteroids.
- Lymphoma and chronic lymphocytic leukaemia.

5.3.3 **Antibody deficiency**

Defective antibody production results in frequent bacterial respiratory infections, often due to encapsulated bacteria (e.g. *Streptococcus pneumoniae*, *Haemophilus influenzae*), or viruses. Causes include:

- Lymphoma and chronic lymphocytic leukaemia
- Multiple myeloma
- Post-HSCT (very prolonged)
- B cell depletion therapy.

5.4 **Clinical features**

Respiratory infection in immunocompromised patients can be severe and progress quickly, so rapid clinical assessment and investigations leading to directed therapy is essential. The presentation varies depending on the patient's immune defect(s) and the pathogen, but includes aysmptomatic radiological infiltrates, fever with no localising symptoms or signs, cough and/or dyspnoea, and fulminant respiratory failure. Few symptoms or signs are specific (e.g. pleural rubs are suggestive of invasive aspergillosis) but the clinical presentation can suggest specific aetiologies as described below (see Table 5.1):

- Onset of cough or dyspnoea over hours or days with pyrexia, high inflammatory markers, and focal radiological changes is likely to represent a bacterial pneumonia
- Subacute onset over days to weeks may suggest opportunistic pathogens, e.g. PCP, viruses or aspergillosis

- Chronic presentation over weeks suggests sub-acute aspergillosis, mycobacterial or *Nocardia* infections or non-infective causes (e.g. organizing pneumonia, pulmonary localization of haematological disease).

As well as the lungs, indwelling line sites, the skin, liver and spleen, and fundi all need to be examined because they may be either the source of the lung infection or sites of secondary spread (e.g. fungal skin lesions or CMV retinitis). An open mind is required so that non-infective causes, atypical presentations of common pathogens, and rarer organisms (e.g. non-*Aspergillus* moulds) are considered, especially in patients who fail to respond to treatment.

Table 5.1 Likely pathogens depending on speed of onset and HRCT appearance

Speed of onset	Pattern of disease on HRCT			
	Consoli-dation	Diffuse ground glass	Nodules (>10 nodules increases chance of mycobacteria or metastatic spread)	Tree in bud (Bronchiolitis)
Acute (days)	Bacterial pneumonia Aspiration	Viral pneumonitis Haemorrhage	Invasive fungi Metastatic infection	Viral bronchiolitis *C. pneumoniae* *M. pneumoniae*
Subacute (days to weeks)	Organizing pneumonia Mycobacteria Invasive fungi *Nocardia* Bacterial pneumonia Aspiration	CMV PCP Drug hypersensitivity	Mycobacteria Invasive fungi *Nocardia* Metastatic infection	Viral bronchiolitis *C. pneumoniae* *M. pneumoniae* *Aspergillus* tracheobronchitis Non TB-mycobacteria
Chronic (weeks)	Organizing pneumonia Mycobacteria *Nocardia* Lymphoma	Drug hypersensitivity	Lymphoma Mycobacteria *Nocardia*	Non TB-mycobacteria Bronchiectasis

5.5 **Radiological presentation**

A chest x-ray is the first investigation but is insensitive in defining the disease pattern, and unless a patient responds rapidly to empirical therapy a CT scan of the lungs is often necessary. CT scans define the radiological presentation precisely, thereby narrowing the differential diagnosis and aiding the selection of empirical therapy, and can identify the lungs as the source of infection in patients with a PUO before x-ray changes are apparent. The main patterns of radiological presentation are discussed below (see Figure 5.1). Mixed or indistinct radiological patterns do occur and in these patients the clinical approach to management will have to be broader and more flexible.

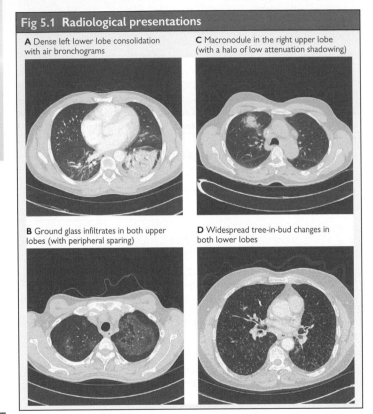

Fig 5.1 Radiological presentations

A Dense left lower lobe consolidation with air bronchograms

C Macronodule in the right upper lobe (with a halo of low attenuation shadowing)

B Ground glass infiltrates in both upper lobes (with peripheral sparing)

D Widespread tree-in-bud changes in both lower lobes

5.5.1 **Consolidation (Figure 5.1A)**

Patches of consolidation in the context of a rapidly developing infection suggest pyogenic bacterial infection, and can be treated after blood and sputum culture with broad-spectrum antibiotics according to local protocols. No response within 48–72 hours should prompt a switch to second-line antibacterial therapy, and bronchoscopy with bronchoalveolar lavage (BAL) should be considered. With less acute clinical presentations, consolidation could also be due to invasive aspergillosis (especially if multiple, wedge-shaped or pleurally-based patches), nocardia, and cryptogenic organizing pneumonia.

Early bronchoscopy is necessary, and percutaneous CT-guided or a VATS biopsy considered if there is no diagnosis or no response to empirical therapy.

5.5.2 Ground glass infiltrates (Figure 5.1B)

Asymmetric pulmonary infiltrates suggest bacterial pneumonia, and can be managed as above. Diffuse largely symmetrical ground glass infiltrates suggest a viral pneumonia or PCP, or non-infective causes (e.g. idiopathic pneumonia syndrome and drug reactions). Nasopharyngeal aspirates (NPA) for respiratory viruses and assessing the patient's CMV status are necessary. If the NPA is negative or the patient has CMV viraemia, bronchoscopy with BAL and perhaps transbronchial biopsy (TBB) should be considered, but these patients are often markedly hypoxic so increasing the risk of bronchoscopy and forcing empirical treatment. VATS biopsy should be considered if there is no diagnosis and a poor response to empirical therapy, but percutaneous biopsy is inappropriate due to the high complication rate (bleeding and pneumothorax).

5.5.3 Nodules (Figure 5.1C)

Nodules can be caused by haematogenous dissemination of bacteria or candida, and can be treated empirically if the patient has an infected indwelling device or candidaemia. Mycobacterial or *Nocardia* infection, or malignant disease are alternative causes of lung nodules, and a small number of macronodules (>2 cm) suggest invasive aspergillosis. Nodules should be investigated by bronchoscopy, and/or percutaneous CT-guided or VATS biopsy, although empirical anti-fungal treatment is an alternative if the patient is at risk for invasive aspergillosis, especially if the halo or crescent signs are present.

5.5.4 Tree-in-bud (Figure 5.1D)

This distinctive CT appearance is suggestive of a bronchiolitis, commonly caused by respiratory viruses in immunosuppressed patients with usually bilateral and symmetrical tree-in-bud changes. *Chlamydophila sp.* or *Mycoplasma sp.* infection are also possible. An NPA is often diagnostic for respiratory viruses, but if negative, bronchscopy and BAL should be considered. Additional causes of tree-in-bud changes include infective exacerbations of underlying bronchiectasis (common post-HSCT or in patients with chronic haematological malignancies), aspergillus tracheobronchitis or mycobacterial infection (focal changes and associated with nodules).

5.6 Other important factors

Additional factors to consider include:
• Previous positive microbiology results

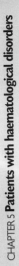

Fig 5.2 Diagnostic algorithm for investigation of new respiratory symptoms in haematology patients

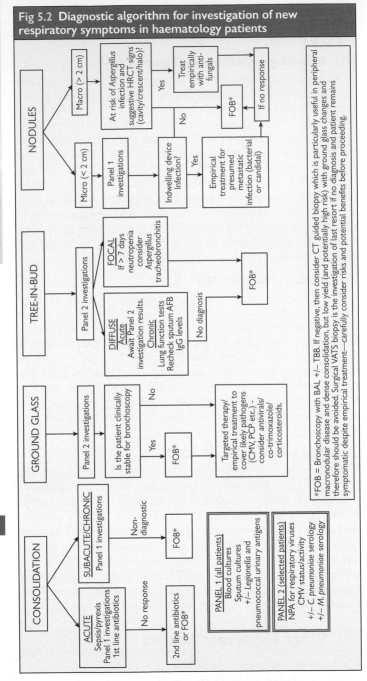

NODULES

Macro (> 2 cm) → At risk of Aspergillus infection and suggestive HRCT signs (cavity/crescent/halo)? → Yes → Treat empirically with anti-fungals → If no response → FOB*

No → FOB*

Micro (< 2 cm) → Panel 1 investigations → Indwelling device Infection? → Yes → Empirical treatment for presumed metastatic infection (bacterial or candidal)

TREE-IN-BUD

Panel 2 investigations

FOCAL
If > 7 days neutropenia consider Aspergillus tracheobronchitis → FOB*

DIFFUSE
Acute
Await Panel 2 investigation results.
Chronic
Lung function tests
Recheck sputum AFB
IgG levels → No diagnosis → FOB*

GROUND GLASS

Panel 2 investigations → Is the patient clinically stable for bronchoscopy → Yes → FOB* → Targeted therapy/ empirical treatment to cover likely pathogens (CMV, PCP etc.) - consider antivirals/ co-trimoxazole/ corticosteroids.

No

CONSOLIDATION

ACUTE
Sepsis/pyrexis
Panel 1 investigations
1st line antibiotics → No response → 2nd line antibiotics or FOB*

SUBACUTE/CHRONIC
Panel 1 investigations → Non-diagnostic → FOB*

PANEL 1 (all patients)
Blood cultures
Sputum cultures
+/– Legionella and pneumococcal urinary antigens

PANEL 2 (selected patients)
NPA for respiratory viruses
CMV status/activity
+/– C. pneumoniae serology
+/– M. pneumoniae serology

*FOB = Bronchoscopy with BAL +/– TBB. If negative, then consider CT guided biopsy which is particularly useful in peripheral macronodular disease and dense consolidation, but low yield (and potentially high risk) with ground glass changes and therefore should be avoided. Surgical VATS biopsy is the investigation of last resort if no diagnosis and patient remains symptomatic despite empirical treatment—carefully consider risks and potential benefits before proceeding.

- Prophylaxis regimens (e.g. co-trimoxazole prophylaxis makes PCP unlikely)
- Local epidemics and contacts with infectious sources (e.g. respiratory viruses)
- Ethnicity and travel (risk of TB or unusual infections)
- Pre-existing lung disease (e.g. cavities at sites of old *Aspergillus* infection that can recur during subsequent episodes of immunosuppression).

5.7 **Investigations**

Which investigations are required depends on the patient's clinical and radiological presentation as discussed above and shown in Figure 5.2. All patients should have:

- Full blood count and white cell differential
- Urea & electrolytes (U&Es, baseline to guide antibiotic therapy options)
- Liver function tests (LFTs, identifies liver or bone as additional sites of infection)
- Inflammatory markers (e.g. a CRP >250 mg/L suggests bacterial infection)
- Chest x-ray
- Sputum, blood, pleural fluid, and urine cultures.

Potential additional investigations include:

- Nasopharyngeal aspirate (NPA) for respiratory viruses
- Legionella and pneumococcal urinary antigen
- Serology for atypical bacteria (probably poor sensitivity in immunosuppressed patients)
- CMV serology and PCR for level of viraemia: identifies patients at risk of CMV pneumonitis
- Serum or BAL galactomannan or glucan antigen testing for fungal pathogens (sensitivity and specificity remains unclear)
- HRCT of the lungs (discussed above).
- Bronchoscopy. Sputum cultures are often negative and bronchoscopy should be considered early for patients who fail to respond to empirical treatment or when fungal or viral opportunistic pathogens are suspected. Bronchoscopy is safe in haematology patients even with thrombocytopenia and has a diagnostic yield of 40–60%, although the sensitivity for *Aspergillus* or PCP is not high enough to exclude these infections by a negative BAL. BAL should be sent for (a) bacterial and fungal culture, (b) cytology and microscopy (*Pneumocystis* cysts, AFBs, Gram staining, CMV, etc.), and (c) antigen, immunofluorescence, or PCR-based tests for CMV and respiratory viruses.

TBB increases the diagnostic yield for ground glass infiltrates by approximately 10%, but is often contraindicated due to thrombocytopenia or dyspnoea.

- CT guided biopsy. Safe and has a high diagnostic yield for macronodules or dense patches of peripheral consolidation (*Aspergillus*, mycobacterial and *Nocardia* infections all have diagnostic histological appearances)
- VATS or open surgical biopsy. The diagnostic intervention of last resort, requires careful consideration of the risks and potential benefits before proceeding.

5.8 **Treatment**

Treatment needs to be started as soon as possible and should cover all the most likely pathogens identified from the clinical evaluation. The treatment options for specific conditions are:

5.8.1 **Bacteria**

Presumed bacterial pneumonia: Broad-spectrum antibiotics to cover Gram positive organisms, coliforms and resistant Gram negative bacteria (e.g. *Pseudomonas*), e.g. broad-spectrum β-lactam +/− an aminoglycoside; follow local guidelines and account for local bacterial resistance patterns. No response within 48–72 hours, switch to second line treatment (e.g. a carbapenem) and consider cover for MRSA or anaerobes. Add a macrolide to treat atypical organisms, such as *Legionella sp.* and *Mycoplasma pneumoniae*, if community acquired infection.

Nocardia: prolonged treatment with co-trimoxazole, β-lactams, or carbapenems.

5.8.2 **Viral infections**

With the exception of CMV and perhaps influenza A, the efficacy of antivirals is poor and treatment is mainly supportive.

CMV: ganciclovir 2.5–5.0mg/kg bd/tds IV or foscarnet 60mg/kg tds IV for 14–21 days.

Influenza A: oseltamivir 75mg bd oral or zanamivir 10mg bd inhaled.

RSV: ribavirin 0.8 mg/kg nebulized over 12 hours or palivizumab 15mg/kg IV (anti-RSV monoclonal antibody).

Adenovirus: cidofovir 1–5mg/kg weekly IV.

5.8.3 **Fungi**

Aspergillus: Voriconazole 4mg/kg per day IV or 200mg bd oral, or caspofungin 50mg od IV, or amphotericin B 1–5mg/kg per day IV or posaconazole 400mg bd oral. Voriconazole and caspofungin are often better tolerated and equal in efficacy to amphotericin B. Treatment is often prolonged.

PCP: co-trimoxazole 120mg/kg/day IV/oral for 3 days in divided doses, then 100 mg/kg daily, or clindamycin 600mg qds IV/oral + primaquine 15–30mg od oral for 21 days (unlicensed in UK) + if hypoxic (PaO$_2$ < 9.3 kPa) prednisolone 40mg bd for 5 days then od for 5 days then 20mg od for 11 days oral.

5.9 **Notes on specific opportunistic pathogens**

5.9.1 **Pulmonary aspergillosis**

- Invasive pulmonary aspergillosis (IPA) is a common and important disease with a high mortality in severely immunosuppressed patients. It usually occurs in patients with prolonged (>10 days) neutropenia, and in patients with graft versus host disease and/or treated with high dose corticosteroids

- *A. fumigatus* causes 70% of cases (the rest mainly *A. flavus*, *A. niger, A. terreus*). Rarer mould infections (*Fusarium*, *Zygomycetes*, *Penicillium, Scedosporium*) have a similar presentation

- Inhaled conidia propagate in the lungs to form hyphae that directly invade lung tissue, and haematogenous spread can occur (e.g. brain, kidney, heart or skin)

- Presentation is generally subacute, with fever, cough, chest pain and haemoptysis. Signs are usually limited and non-specific, but a pleural rub can occur

- HRCT demonstrates irregular consolidation, cavitation and/or macronodules. Changes specific to IPA include the halo sign (low attenuation surrounding a nodule—occurs within the first week of infection) and the air crescent sign (partial cavitation causing a crescent of air within a nodule—a late sign occurring after three weeks)

- Diagnosis is often clinical, e.g. fever or cough in a neutropenic patient with typical CT appearances, and this can be enough to initiate treatment. Microbiological confirmation can be obtained by BAL (sensitivity 50%) or antigen testing for serum galactomannan or glucan (cell wall constituents, may give false positive results). Percutaneous CT guided biopsy can be helpful (sensitivity 70%) as *Aspergillus* has a distinctive morphology (dichotomous branching hyphae)

- Other forms of invasive aspergillosis include:
  - *Aspergillus* tracheobronchitis. Affects the same patients as IPA, but infection is within the tracheobrochial tree. Causes an unremitting cough, and the CT will show bronchial wall thickening, nodules and focal areas of tree-in-bud changes. Bronchoscopy shows distinctive areas of ulceration with

yellow slough within the bronchial tree, culture and biopsy of which are positive for *Aspergillus*

– Chronic necrotizing pulmonary aspergillosis (CNPA). *Aspergillus* lung infection in patients with lesser degrees of immunosuppression (e.g. corticosteroids, diabetes, structural lung disease). The presentation is with chronic cough, malaise and a slowly (weeks and months) expanding lung mass that may cavitate. The differential diagnosis is cancer and TB, and confirming the diagnosis is often difficult. In contrast to IPA antibodies to *Aspergillus* are frequently positive, but the gold standard is demonstration by histology of fungal hyphae invading lung tissue. Treatment is with prolonged use of antifungal agents and surgical excision if possible, but mortality is high.

5.9.2 **PCP (also see Section 4.3)**

- A fungal infection mainly affecting patients with defects in cell-mediated immunity
- Presents with cough and progressive breathlessness over days and weeks. Oxygen desaturation on exercise is characteristic. CT scans classically show symmetrical ground glass shadowing, mainly in the upper lobes with peripheral sparing
- Diagnosis is often clinical but is confirmed by demonstration of *Pneumocystis* cysts in BAL or induced sputum
- Recurrence after completion of a treatment course can occur, and prophylaxis with co-trimoxazole is usually given (480mg od or 960mg 3 per week).

5.9.3 **Respiratory viruses**

- Parainfluenza, RSV, influenza, adenovirus, metapneumovirus, rhinoviruses
- Mainly affect patients with defects in cell-mediated immunity, and can spread between patients

- Presents with cough, breathlessness, and fever (often low grade). On examination there may be few signs, but inspiratory squeaks are characteristic. CT scan often shows tree-in-bud changes and patches of ground glass infiltrates
- Often persist for weeks in immunosuppressed patients, and can cause respiratory failure and/or significant airway obstruction
- Diagnosis is made with immunofluorescence or PCR on NPA or BAL samples, but treatment options are often limited
- *C. pneumoniae* and *M. pneumoniae* bronchiolitis can have a similar presentation.

5.9.4 **Cytomegalovirus (CMV)**

- Common in patients with defects in cell-mediated immunity
- CMV pneumonitis causes gradual onset of cough, breathlessness, hypoxia and fever, and the CT scan usually shows diffuse ground glass infiltrates
- A diagnosis of CMV pneumonitis requires a significant CMV viraemia. However respiratory infiltrates in patients with CMV viraemia are not necessarily due to a CMV pneumonitis: this is more likely if there is high viral load or this has increased rapidly. BAL can confirm CMV pneumonitis ('owl's eyes' intranuclear inclusions or positive antigen tests, PCR or viral culture)
- Has a high mortality.

5.9.5 **Nocardia species (gram positive, weakly acid-fast filamentous bacteria)**

- Uncommon: affects patients with defects in cell-mediated immunity
- Usually subacute presentation similar in appearance to mycobacterial or fungal disease (macronodules or patches of consolidation that may cavitate)
- Pleural involvement and metastatic spread to other organs are common
- Diagnosed by histological or microbiological examination
- Treat for up to a year. Usually sensitive to co-trimoxazole, β-lactams, cephalosporins, and carbapenems.

Further reading

Brown J.S. (2008) Pneumonia in the non-HIV immunocompromised host. In *Clinical Respiratory Medicine*; Albert R., Spiro S. and Jett J. (eds). Elsevier.

de la Hoz R.E., Stephens G., Sherlock C. (2002) Diagnosis and treatment approaches of CMV infection in adult patients. *Journal of Clinical Virology* **25**(25): S1–S12.

de Pauw B., Walsh T.J., Donnelly J.P., *et al.* (2008) Revised definitions of invasive fungal disease from the European Organization for Research and Treatment of Cancer/Invasive Fungal Infections Cooperative Group and the National Institute of Allergy and Infectious Diseases Mycoses Study Group (EORTC/MSG) Consensus Group. *Clinical infectious diseases: an official publication of the Infectious Diseases Society of America.* **46**(12):1813–21.

Ison M., Hayden F.G. (2002) Viral infections in immunocompromised patients: what's new with respiratory viruses? *Current Opinion in Infectious Diseases* **15**: 355–67.

Maschmeyer G., Beinert T., Buchheidt D., *et al.* (2003) Diagnosis and antimicrobial therapy of pulmonary infiltrates in febrile neutropenic patients. *Ann Hematol* **82**(2): S118–S126.

O'Brien S.N., Blijlevens N.M., Mahfouz T.H., Anaissie E.J. (2003) Infections in patients with hematological cancer: recent developments. *Hematology*: 438–72.

Rañó A., Agusti C., Jiminez P., *et al.* (2001) Pulmonary infiltrates in non-HIV immunocompromised patients: a diagnostic approach using non-invasive and bronchoscopic procedures. *Thorax* **56**: 379–87.

Mayaud C., Cadranel J. (2000). A persistent challenge: the diagnosis of respiratory disease in the non-AIDS immunocompromised host. *Thorax* **55**: 511–17.

Walsh T.J., Anaissie E.J., Denning D.W., *et al.* (2008) Treatment of aspergillosis: clinical practice guidelines of the *Infectious Diseases Society of America. Clinical Journal of Infectious Diseases 1*; **46**(3): 327–60.

Chapter 6

Pleural infections

Clare Hooper and Nick Maskell

Key points

- Pleural infection is associated with a mortality rate of 15–20%
- The bacteriology of community acquired pleural infection is distinct from that of community acquired pneumonia. Empirical antibiotics should always cover penicillin resistant aerobes and anaerobic organisms
- Hospital acquired pleural infection has a worse prognosis than community acquired pleural infection and is most often due to MRSA or gram negative bacteria
- All parapneumonic effusions >1cm in depth should be sampled and fluid pH measured unless frank pus is obtained
- No presenting clinical, biochemical or radiological features accurately predict outcome or the need for surgical intervention, so that early intravenous antibiotics and chest tube drainage with assiduous clinical monitoring for primary treatment failure should be applied to every patient
- Mortality is greater in the elderly and those with co-morbid illnesses. Therefore, they in particular should be considered early for limited surgical drainage procedures if failing to respond to medical management
- Follow up for at least 3 months is mandatory to detect the minority of patients who relapse with pleural sepsis or persistent breathlessness due to pleural thickening.

The incidence of pleural infection is increasing with approximately 13,000 patients diagnosed in the UK each year. Bacterial pleural infection is associated with significant morbidity and carries a mortality of up to 20%; a figure that has not decreased over the past 30 years, despite notable advances in imaging techniques and cardiothoracic surgery.

6.1 **Epidemiology**

While it is most common in the paediatric and elderly population, pleural infection can occur at any age and affects men twice as frequently as women. Clear predisposing factors can be identified in two thirds of patients, with the remainder occurring in previously healthy individuals. Recent series have reported a particularly strong association with diabetes mellitus which is present in more than 20% of patients. Box 6.1 summarizes commonly recognized risk factors.

Box 6.1 Risk factors for pleural infection

Diabetes mellitus
Immunosupression (corticosteroids, chemotherapy, myelosupression etc.)
Gastro-oesophogeal reflux disease*
Alcohol excess
Intravenous drug use
Pleural procedures and thoracic surgery (iatrogenic pleural infection)
Penetrating chest trauma
Intra-abdominal sepsis (sub-phrenic collection)
Bacteraemia
Oesophageal surgery or perforation
Aspiration*
Poor oral hygiene/poor dentition*
*associated with anaerobic pleural infection

6.2 **Pathophysiology and bacteriology**

Bacterial infection of the pleural space may occur as a sequelae of pneumonia, seemingly spontaneously in the absence of parenchymal infection (so called 'primary empyema'), or following a breach of the pleura (in oesophageal rupture, penetrating chest wall trauma or as an iatrogenic phenomenon following thoracic surgery, chest drain placement or pleural aspiration without asepsis). This range of origins is reflected in the bacteriology of pleural infection which is quite distinct from that of community acquired pneumonia; a fact that should be recognized in empirical antibiotic choices.

The microbiological data obtained from the Multicentre Intrapleural Streptokinase Trial (MIST 1) represents the largest series of its kind and provides a sound foundation for our understanding of the bacteriology of modern pleural infection (see Table 6.1). In community acquired disease, *Streptococcus sp.* are responsible in around 50% with *Staphylococcus sp.*, anaerobic organisms, and gram negative bacteria accounting for the other half. Anaerobic organisms are involved in at least 25% of cases, frequently co-existing with aerobes (often *Streptococcus milleri* group) but never in combination with *Streptococcus pneumoniae*. The MIST 1 data confirms that bacteria that are not usually found in community acquired pneumonia, are present in at least 30% of pleural infections. The route of these organisms to the pleural space is poorly understood; an oropharyngeal source with bacteraemia and preferential seeding of the pleura is one possible explanation.

Importantly, atypical organisms such as *Legionella sp.* and *Mycoplasma sp.* very rarely cause pleural infection and were not identified at all in the MIST 1 cohort.

Hospital acquired pleural infection has clearly different microbiology and should be considered a separate disease entity to community acquired infection. *Staphylococcus sp.* (the majority of which are MRSA, accounting for 25% of all positive cultures) and gram negative organisms dominate.

Fungal infection of the pleural space is very rare and carries a poor prognosis, usually occurring in the immunosuppressed or as a secondary infection in those with a chest drain *in situ*.

The spectrum of pathological and radiological changes seen at different stages in bacterial pleural infection is best understood by considering the disease when it originates from pneumonia. About 50–60% of pneumonias are complicated by an exudative pleural effusion which forms as a reactive phenomenon due to increased capillary permeability and the production of pro-inflammatory cytokines, particularly IL-8 and TNF–α. In simple parapneumonic effusions, pleural fluid has a normal alkaline pH, a glucose equivalent to that in the blood, and is culture negative. In most cases parapneumonic effusions resolve with antibiotics alone.

Four per cent of parapneumonic effusions progress to pleural infection. Bacterial translocation across inflamed visceral pleura amplifies the immune response within the pleural space with chemotaxis of neutrophils into pleural fluid and the activation of the coagulation cascade resulting in fibrin deposition over both the visceral and parietal pleura and the formation of septae within the effusion. At this stage, the 'early fibrinopurulent phase', pleural fluid has a high LDH, low pH (≤ 7.2) and low glucose due to increased metabolic activity by bacteria and inflammatory cells within the pleural space. Pleural fluid may be frankly purulent (confirming an 'empyema'), serous, bloody or turbid.

Finally, in the organising phase or 'late fibrinopurulent phase', fibroblast proliferation results in the formation of a pleural 'peel' which sometimes causes restriction in lung function and produces a persistent cavity, encouraging re-accumulation of infected fluid after initial tube drainage.

Progression through these stages varies between patients and delay in presentation with pleural infection does not imply inevitability of pleural thickening or a higher likelihood of primary medical treatment failure.

Table 6.1 Summarized bacteriology data from the MIST 1 cohort. All bacterial isolates obtained from pleural fluid and blood cultures and pleural fluid PCR

Bacteria	Community acquired cases Number of isolates (% total isolates)	Nosocomial cases Number of isolates (% total isolates)
Aerobes		
Streptococcus sp.	176 (52%)	11 (18%)
Streptococcus milleri group	80	4
Streptococcus pneumoniae	71	3
Streptococcus pyogenes	9	0
Other *Streptococcal sp.*	16	4
Staphyloccocus sp.	35 (10%)	21 (35%)
Staphylococcus aureus	27	6
MRSA	7	15
Staphylococcus epidermidis	1	0
Enterococcus sp.	4 (1%)	7 (12%)
Gram negative bacteria	29 (9%)	14 (23%)
Escherichia coli	11	2
Other coliforms	4	6
Proteus sp.	6	2
Enterobacter sp.	5	1
Pseudomonas aeruginosa	3	3
Anaerobes	67 (20%)	5 (8%)
Fusobacterium	19	1
Bacteroides sp.	16	1
Peptostreptococcus sp.	9	0
Prevotella sp.	13	1
Other anaerobes	10	2
Other bacteria	23 (6%)	2 (3%)
Total	336	60

6.3 **Diagnosis and investigations**

Many patients present with clinical signs and chest x-ray evidence of a pleural effusion accompanied by systemic sepsis. Additionally, pleural infection should be suspected in patients with pneumonia when clinical features of infection do not settle despite adequate antibiotics. In pneumonia, failure of the C-reactive protein (CRP) level to fall on day 3 to 50% of its value at presentation is associated with a greater likelihood of empyema.

Distinguishing pleural infection from pleural malignancy is a common dilemma, and given the divergent optimum investigation and management pathways of the 2 conditions, involvement of an experienced physician at an early stage is sensible. Pleural fluid pH does not distinguish pleural infection from other causes, as pleural acidosis is also common in malignancy and inflammatory pleuritis (e.g. rheumatoid effusion). A differential pleural fluid cell count is often the most useful test when there is diagnostic doubt, with neutrophil predominance indicating bacterial infection and lymphocyte predominance being found in a host of other conditions including malignancy, cardiac failure and tuberculosis. Serum biomarkers such as procalcitonin may prove useful in the early differentiation of pleural infection from malignancy and trials examining this are underway.

If the clinical suspicion is of sepsis, management for pleural infection in the first instance is appropriate while pleural fluid tests and imaging are awaited.

6.4 Imaging

A pleural effusion may be clearly evident on chest x-ray and parenchymal consolidation may also be visible. Loculated pleural fluid frequently produces a smooth sub-pleural opacity (Figure 6.1) which can be mistaken for a parenchymal mass. Chest x-ray appearances may be difficult to interpret and if there is clinical suspicion of pleural infection, a thoracic ultrasound scan is a sensitive and specific means of confirming and locating pleural fluid and is required to guide pleural aspiration.

Appearances on ultrasound (Figure 6.2) reflect the stage of organization of the pleural infection but do not predict outcome. Pleural fluid may appear anechoic, septated, homogenously echogenic, or have a complex non-septated appearance. Ultrasound is the most sensitive means of detecting fluid septation and loculation.

CT scans are not required for all cases of pleural infection but are useful if initial drainage is incomplete with persisting sepsis and chest x-ray abnormalities. Contrast enhanced CT is useful to distinguish pleural infection from pulmonary abscess, to demonstrate underlying mass lesions, oesophageal rupture and plan cardiothoracic surgical procedures. When pleural infection has entered the organizing phase, the pleura enhances brightly with contrast (Figure 6.3) and suspended air bubbles may be seen within infected pleural fluid reflecting loculation.

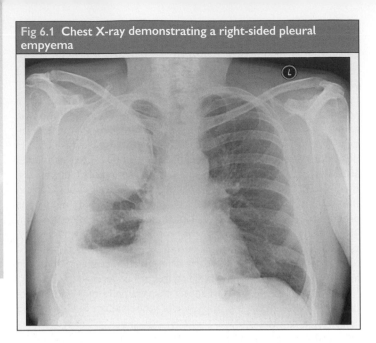

Fig 6.1 Chest X-ray demonstrating a right-sided pleural empyema

CT identifies the position of existing chest tubes and demonstrates the distribution of pleural fluid and thickening, guiding the placement of subsequent drains or indicating a low likelihood of success with percutaneous drainage and the need for surgical referral.

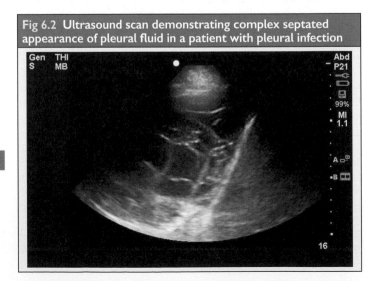

Fig 6.2 Ultrasound scan demonstrating complex septated appearance of pleural fluid in a patient with pleural infection

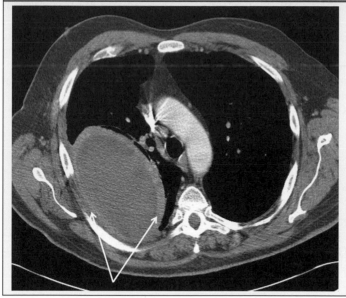

Fig 6.3 **Pleural phase contrast CT scan demonstrating a right empyema with bright enhancement of the thickened parietal and visceral pleural (indicated by arrows)—'split pleura' sign**

6.5 **Pleural fluid analysis**

Pleural aspiration can be particularly challenging in pleural infection due to the potential for loculation and pleural thickening. Bedside ultrasound is essential to improve the likelihood of success and avoid organ trauma. The appearance of pleural fluid should be recorded.
   Pleural fluid should be sent for:

- Microscopy and culture (sending both plain and blood culture bottles increases yield, particularly for anaerobic organisms)
- pH (if not purulent. Blood gas syringe and machine should be used. Avoid exposure of fluid to air or lignocaine)
- Protein and LDH (if not purulent)
- Cytology with differential cell count
- AFB and TB culture (where there is particular suspicion of TB).

Blood cultures should always be sent at presentation as they increase the chance of a positive microbiological diagnosis above culturing pleural fluid alone.

6.6 **Pleural fluid pH**

The most reliable indicator of the need for tube drainage for adequate resolution of sepsis in a parapneumonic effusion is a pleural fluid pH of ≤7.2 which implies progression to pleural infection. This cutoff is a useful practical guide, but as a small number of patients with a pH of >7.2 do go on to develop pleural infection requiring intervention, the value should be interpreted carefully in clinical context. The following should be considered when interpreting pleural fluid pH:

- Variations in sample collection technique have a clinically significant impact on measured pleural fluid pH. Most importantly, small volumes of residual lignocaine in the needle or syringe significantly reduces pH and exposure of pleural fluid to air increases it
- The measured pH of different pleural fluid locules can be highly variable
- Pleural infection due to *Proteus sp.* is associated with an alkaline pH as the bacteria splits ammonia to form urea.

Other indications for chest tube drainage in parapneumonic effusions are summarised in Box 6.2.

Box 6.2 Indications for chest tube drainage in patients presenting with signs of sepsis and a pleural effusion

- Pleural fluid pH ≤7.2
- Pleural fluid frankly purulent
- Positive pleural fluid Gram stain or culture
- Loculation on ultrasound scan
- Very large parapneumonic effusion with respiratory compromise

---

6.7 **Management**

After confirmation of the diagnosis of pleural infection, rapid treatment with appropriate empirical antibiotics, and chest tube drainage followed by continuous reassessment of the need for thoracic surgical intervention is essential.

6.8 **Antibiotics**

Early antibiotic therapy for community acquired pleural infection must cover penicillin resistant aerobes and commonly isolated anaerobes.

Suitable regimes include penicillins combined with β-lactamase inhibitors (e.g. co-amoxiclav). In penicillin allergy, clindamycin alone can be used for its broad spectrum activity. These antibiotics appear to have reasonable penetration to the pleural space in contrast to aminoglycosides which should be avoided. Coverage for atypical pathogens, such as *Legionella sp.* or *Mycoplasma sp.*, with macrolide antibiotics is unnecessary.

Positive microbiology is ultimately obtained from pleural fluid or blood cultures in 60% to 70% of cases of pleural infection and once available, should be used to guide therapy. Anaerobic organisms are particularly difficult to culture and frequently co-exist with *S. milleri*. Nucleic acid amplification testing (PCR) applied to pleural fluid was shown to significantly increase the number of anaerobic isolates in the MIST1 cohort. However, as this test is not routinely available, it is sensible to continue with anaerobic antibiotic cover empirically even if aerobic organisms have been isolated. A caveat to this is that anaerobes have not been shown to co-exist with *S. pneumoniae* so that when this is cultured, single agent treatment with benzylpenicillin is adequate.

Treatment for hospital acquired infection, should reflect the increased incidence of gram negative organisms and MRSA seen in these patients. Vancomycin in combination with piperacillin/tazobactam or a carbopenem represents a good combination in this setting.

There is little robust evidence to guide the route or duration of antibiotics, but conventionally, intravenous therapy is given for at least the first 5 days and oral antibiotics continued for a further 2 to 4 weeks with the duration determined by clinical and biochemical progress as well as radiological resolution of the pleural collection.

6.9 **Chest tube drainage**

Chest drains should be placed with bedside ultrasound guidance. Success of tube drainage is determined by infected fluid viscosity, degree of loculation and patency of the chest tube. There is no evidence to support the use of large bore over small bore tubes (10–14F) which can be inserted using a Seldinger technique and are more comfortable for patients. Flushing with 20–30 ml sterile saline 3–4 times a day with continuous suction (up to −20 cm H_2O) may help to maintain patency of small bore tubes and is usual practice in some centres.

Timing of drain removal is usually guided by cessation of fluid drainage, radiological resolution and improvement in clinical and blood markers of sepsis. Further imaging with contrast enhanced CT is indicated if sepsis fails to resolve and there is evidence of a residual pleural fluid collection. This allows identification of underlying obstructing mass lesions and the distribution of fluid and pleural thickening.

While the most important randomized controlled trial of single agent intrapleural fibrinolysis in pleural infection (MIST 1) did not demonstrate a significant improvement in outcomes, results of the 2011 MIST 2 trial suggest that a combination of intrapleural fibrinolysis (specifically tissue plasminogen activator (t-PA)) and DNase may be effective in augmenting pleural fluid drainage and reducing surgical referral rates. In this 210 patient RCT, patients randomized to t-PA and DNase were shown to have significantly improved chest x-ray clearance, 77% fewer surgical referrals and a mean of 6.7 fewer in-patient days when compared to placebo. It is proposed that the combination of breakdown of fibrinous loculations and reduction in fluid viscosity achieved by the two agents improves overall drainage. Single agent therapy alone did not significantly improve outcomes and DNase mono-therapy appeared to increase surgical referral rates and is probably harmful.

Thus, dual therapy with t-PA and DNase may provide a useful option for patients who are unfit for surgery in the future but further larger studies are required to confirm these promising results before adoption in common clinical practice.

6.10 **General management points**

Patients with pleural infection should receive specialist respiratory care in light of the high mortality associated with the condition, the potential for diagnostic uncertainty, complexities of timing and case selection for surgical intervention and the need for assiduous follow-up over a minimum of 3 months following presentation (late recurrence after initial resolution of sepsis is not uncommon).

Hypoalbuminaemia and poor nutrition before and during the acute illness are poor prognostic factors in pleural infection and nutritional supplementation should therefore be initiated at diagnosis and early consideration given to nasogastric feeding.

Patients are at increased risk of thromboembolic disease and should receive thrombosis prophylaxis during their inpatient stay.

6.11 **Thoracic surgery for pleural infection**

It is unclear at what stage surgical intervention produces a better outcome above continued medical management in patients with pleural infection. It would seem feasible that late fibrinopurulent and organizing stage pleural infection is most likely to require surgery for complete resolution, but it is well documented that many patients in this category recover without such invasive intervention. Depth of pleural thickening on initial CT scan is also a poor predictor of need for surgery. Thick pleural peel frequently resolves over the weeks following discharge if sepsis has not necessitated surgery.

It is common practice to seek a surgical opinion when sepsis has failed to improve after 5 days of appropriate antibiotics and chest tube drainage, or earlier in patients presenting with significant pleural collections where an adequate drain position cannot be achieved because of extensive loculation. Decisions regarding early surgical referral are founded on individual clinical judgement, age, co-morbid illnesses and patient preference. Operative mortality is clearly higher for the elderly and frail but as this group are the most likely to die as a result of pleural infection (see Figure 6.4), there is a particularly compelling argument for referring them early for limited surgical drainage procedures under local anaesthetic.

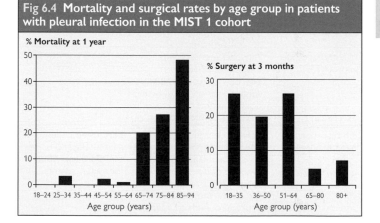

Fig 6.4 Mortality and surgical rates by age group in patients with pleural infection in the MIST 1 cohort

Table 6.2 summarizes common surgical approaches in the management of pleural infection. The choice of surgical procedure varies according to local thoracic surgery experience and preference, anatomical distribution of pleural infection, and patient fitness.

For patients who are unfit for or decline even limited surgical drainage procedures, the placement of multiple small-bore chest drains under image guidance in an attempt to drain as many locules of infected fluid as possible thereby reducing systemic sepsis, should be considered.

69

6.12 **Prognosis and outcome**

Unfortunately, no presenting clinical, radiological or pleural fluid characteristics have been shown to reliably predict prognosis or indicate the need for early surgical referral. All patients should therefore be managed with the same systematic and vigilant approach.

Table 6.2 Surgical management of pleural infection		
Procedure	**Details**	**Advantages**
Video assisted thoracoscopic surgery (VATS) with pleural debridement.	Now the most frequently employed approach. Achieves complete clearance of infected pleural tissue and fluid in most cases. Late stage organisation appears to increase risk of failure and subsequent need for thoracotomy and decortication.	Minimally invasive. Short operation and recovery times. Acceptable cosmesis. May be done (although infrequently) under local anaesthetic and sedation.
Thoracotomy and decortication.	Traditional approach. Successful clearance of infected tissue in 90% of cases. Major operation requiring general anaesthetic. Most patients have some surgical site pain for at least 12 months.	Highest success rates in fit patients. Effective pleural space clearance in advanced empyema (late decortication).
Mini-thoracotomy with VATS.	A hybrid approach with advantages of both procedures but a smaller surgical incision and shorter operation time than traditional thoracotomy.	
Rib resection and open drainage.	Limited clearance procedure which can be VATS assisted and leads to open drainage of the pleural space into a bag or drain for several months after the procedure. Aims to address sepsis rather than pleural thickening.	Performed under local anaesthetic and is therefore appropriate for frailer patients.

The presence of frank pleural pus, delayed presentation and pleural fluid loculation have been suggested (but not consistently) to be associated with an adverse outcome or utility in guiding management decisions in published series.

Hospital acquired infection has a worse outcome, perhaps due to its microbiology as well as the baseline co-morbid illness of the patients.

Mean mortality rates of 15 to 20% in the 12 months following presentation have been reported in recent series, with the majority of deaths occurring in those over 65 years of age.

Further reading

Davies C.W., Kearney S.E., Gleeson F.V., Davies R.J.O. (1999) Predictors of outcome and long-term survival in patients with pleural infection. *Am J Respir Crit Care Med* **160**:1682–7.

Davies H.E., Davies R.J.O, Davies C.W.H. (2009) The British Thoracic Society Guidelines for the management of pleural infection. *Thorax* (In press).

Heffner E., Brown L.K., Barbieri C., DeLeo J.M. (1995) Pleural fluid chemistry in parapneumonic effusions. A meta-analysis. *Am J Crit Care Med* **151**:1700–08.

Maskell N.A., Davies C.W.H., Nunn A.J., *et al.* (2005) UK controlled trial of intrapleural streptokinase for pleural infection. *N Eng J Med* **352**: 865–74.

Maskell N.A., Batt S., Hedley E.L., Davies C.W.H., Gillespie S.H., Davies R.J.O. (2006) The bacteriology of pleural infection by genetic and standard methods and its mortality significance. *Am J Respir Crit Care Med* **174**: 817–23.

Rahman NM (2011) Intrapleural use of Tissue Plasminogen Activator and DNase in Pleural Infection. *N Engl J Med*; **365**: 518–26.

Chapter 7

Influenza and other respiratory viral infections

Jonathan S. Nguyen-Van-Tam

Key points

- Although respiratory infections in temperate zones occur year round, their distribution is highly seasonal with a consistent winter peak in both northern and southern temperate zones
- It is not possible to accurately assign a specific respiratory viral aetiology to any set of presenting clinical symptoms and signs; surveillance data are useful to determine when influenza activity is widespread
- The timing and intensity of influenza activity each winter is highly variable but, once present, activity tends to persist for 8–10 weeks
- Influenza infections occur year round, and out-of-season activity is not infrequently detected in schools and residential homes for the elderly (the diagnostic possibility cannot be excluded simply because elderly residents have been vaccinated)
- In the treatment of influenza, both oseltamivir and zanamivir are licensed to be started within 48 hours of symptom onset
- If influenza is suspected and antiviral therapy deemed appropriate, this should not be deferred pending virological confirmation, because early instigation improves outcomes
- Hospital practitioners confronted with a patient with suspected or proven influenza, who is severely unwell, should not hesitate to start therapy >48 hours after symptom onset, nor to continue this for >5 days
- In patients with confirmed influenza who are unresponsive to antiviral therapy, consider the possibility of resistance and the need to switch drugs.

7.1 **Burden of disease and recognition**

The burden of illness due to respiratory viral infections is immense. Each year in the UK, respiratory conditions account for roughly one quarter of all primary care consultations. The vast majority of these arise because of a respiratory infection, and of those due to infection, the commonest aetiology is a respiratory virus. Although respiratory viral infections occur year round, their distribution is highly seasonal with a consistent winter peak in both northern and southern temperate zones. This is clearly illustrated in the UK by the variation in 'cold or flu' calls to the NHS Direct telephone advisory service according to the time of year (Figure 7.1); indeed it has been estimated that up to 50% of this seasonal variation can be accounted for by influenza and respiratory syncytial virus (RSV) activity alone. In addition to seasonal variation, the incidence of respiratory viral infections is strongly age-related, being generally much commoner among children, especially those in pre-school and primary age groups.

Fig 7.1 Weekly NHS Direct 'cold/flu' calls (as a % of total NHS Direct calls) against weekly laboratory reports for influenza, respiratory syncytial virus, parainfluenza virus and rhinovirus

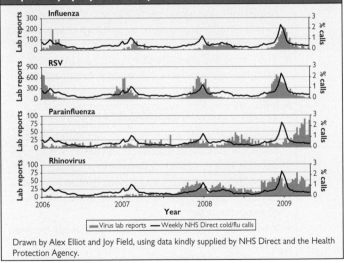

Drawn by Alex Elliot and Joy Field, using data kindly supplied by NHS Direct and the Health Protection Agency.

A considerable range of clinical syndromes is associated with acute respiratory viral infection including upper and lower respiratory tract infections (URTI and LRTI). Those for which the commonest cause is a respiratory virus are listed in Table 7.1.

While respiratory viral infection may be caused by over 200 distinct virus types, certain ones are of central importance, either due to their frequency, severity, novelty, or public health impact. These are listed in Table 7.2.

Table 7.1 Clinical syndromes for which the commonest cause is a respiratory virus

URTI	LRTI
common cold	bronchitis
influenza-like illness (ILI)	influenza-like illness (ILI)
tonsillitis	laryngotracheobronchitis (croup)
otitis media	bronchiolitis
sinusitis	
laryngitis	
sore throat	

*influenza-like illness may affect both parts of the respiratory tree

Table 7.2 Important respiratory viral infections in humans

Virus	Reason for importance
Rhinoviruses	The commonest respiratory viral infection.
Coronaviruses	The second commonest respiratory virus infection.
Adenoviruses	Especially common in children <2 years; an important cause of viral pneumonia
Influenza viruses (types A & B)	Associated with epidemics (A and B) and pandemics (A only); excess mortality and morbidity well described; major seasonal impact in elderly and persons with chronic illness; effective drugs for treatment and prophylaxis; also vaccine preventable.
Parainfluenza viruses	Types 1 and 2 (Para 1, Para 2) principle causes of croup in young children; type 3 (Para 3) important cause of bronchiolitis and pneumonia in children <6 months.
Respiratory syncytial virus (RSV)	The commonest cause of bronchiolitis and pneumonia in infants and young children; nosocomial spread is well documented; immunoprophylaxis is possible (palivizumab); vaccine is badly needed but not yet available.
Human metapneumovirus (hMPV)	Novel pathogen, first isolated in 2001. Burden of illness in humans not yet fully established but probably most important in children <5 years.
SARS coronavirus (SARS-CoV)	Novel human pathogen responsible for >8000 cases of respiratory illness of whom almost 10% died, between late 2002 and summer 2003. Spread rapidly across the globe and was a pandemic 'near-miss'. Threat has currently receded, but disease not considered to have been eradicated.

Although certain respiratory viruses are more commonly associated with certain clinical syndromes, e.g. RSV with croup and bronchiolitis in children and acute bronchitis in adults, assigning presenting clinical symptoms and signs to a specific viral aetiology is an inexact science. Similarly, 'old wives tales' associated with the identification of specific viral infections, e.g. 'you know when you've got real influenza because you can't get out of bed' are equally unhelpful in disentangling virus aetiology. Some data exist which suggest that influenza is more likely than other respiratory viruses to precipitate medical consultation but, even so, there is good evidence to suggest that about 50% of all influenza infections are asymptomatic; clinical illness tends to range from mild to severe for most if not all respiratory viruses. This is not to say that respiratory viral infections are always indistinguishable. For example, influenza is said to be recognizable by its particularly abrupt onset; but it is often difficult without virological testing.

Although clinical diagnoses tend to be somewhat non-specific, it can rightly be argued that identification of the precise virus aetiology does not usually affect the clinical management of an individual patient because most treatment is only supportive. Thus the vast majority of acute respiratory infections, assumed to be of viral aetiology, are not investigated in the community or in hospital, despite the fact that modern laboratory methods, based on multiplex PCR, can screen rapidly for a panel of common respiratory viruses. These techniques are often only applied systematically during research studies and in a few reference laboratories or centres of excellence.

Of all human respiratory virus infections, influenza is easily the most important. Through a combination of regular (winter) seasonal epidemics and occasional pandemics, the total morbidity and mortality inflicted by the virus is immense. In recent years, even greater attention has been focused on this particular virus due to the human health threat posed by avian and animal influenzas, most notably influenza A/H5N1 and A/H7N7, and by the emergence of a novel pandemic virus of swine origin (influenza A/H1N1) in Spring 2009. Despite the generally mild nature of the 2009 pandemic, a small proportion of fatal or life-threatening infections ensued and critical care capacity came under sustained pressure in many parts of the world (Box 7.1). The 2009 pandemic virus replaced the previous seasonal A/H1N1 virus and became a post-pandemic seasonal virus, circulating alongside A/H3N2 and influenza B. Indeed, significant activity due to A/H1N1 occurred during the immediate post-pandemic winter season in Britain in 2010–11.

An additional feature which increases the public health importance and clinical significance of influenza compared with other respiratory viruses is that it is the only respiratory virus infection for which preventive and specific treatments are both available. It is therefore

Box 7.1 2009 Pandemic influenza (A/H1N1)

- First cases and possible epicentre in Mexico, March 2009
- Rapid global spread, leading to WHO pandemic declaration, 11 June 2009
- Triple-reassortant influenza A/H1N1 virus of mainly swine origin
- Two waves in UK (Spring 2009 and Autumn/Winter 2009–10)
- Typical symptoms, comparable with seasonal influenza, but raised incidence of gastrointestinal disturbance
- Generally mild, self-limiting illness, with highest incidence in children and young adults
- People >60 years of relatively spared due to past exposure to antigenically similar viruses in early life
- Case fatality rate 0.03 to 0.05%, but 90% of all deaths in people under 65 years
- Low excess mortality overall, but broadly similar in impact to 1968–69 pandemic in terms of years of life lost
- Despite low hospitalisation rate (0.5 to 1%), around 20% of hospitalised cases required intensive care (severe hypoxaemia, ARDS and renal failure) of whom about 25% died – health capacity pressures greatest in critical care settings
- Risk factors for poor outcome as for seasonal influenza, including very strong signal for increased risk in pregnancy
- Severe/morbid obesity identified as new risk factor for severe outcome
- Monovalent pandemic vaccines available from October2009
- Neuraminidase inhibitors widely used; analyses suggest that early use linked to lower risk of severe outcome – mainly low levels of resistance.
- WHO declared pandemic ended, 10 August 2010

unsurprising that surveillance schemes for the detection of influenza are much more well-developed than for other viruses. In the UK, several primary care sentinel schemes based on clinical consultations are in operation each winter, of which some are also linked to virological sampling. These linked data are especially valuable. However there are no similar systems routinely in place in hospitals, and consequently the burden of hospital admissions due to respiratory viral infection is poorly understood at the present time. Nevertheless, individual hospital studies focussing on community-acquired pneumonia and acute medical admissions have identified that respiratory viral infections are associated with many more hospital admissions than recognized routinely in clinical practice. In addition they are associated with non-respiratory admissions (e.g. cardiac conditions and diabetes) and are a well-recognised and common cause of exacerbations of asthma and COPD.

7.2 **Influenza management**

Influenza presents as an acute illness characterized by cough, malaise, and feverishness (in >80% of clinically recognised cases), typically of rapid onset. Other additional symptoms (in order of frequency) are: (in 50-79% of cases) chills, headache, anorexia, coryza, myalgia, and sore throat; (<50%) sputum, dizziness, hoarseness, chest pain; (<10%) vomiting and diarrhoea. In reality recognition of influenza should be made by combining clinical judgement with information from surveillance schemes about the circulation of influenza in the community.

The timing and intensity of influenza activity each winter is highly variable but, once present, activity tends to persist for 8–10 weeks. Usually one virus dominates but at the present time influenza A/H3N2, A/H1N1, and influenza B are all encountered to some extent each winter. Influenza A activity tends to begin before the turn of the year whereas influenza B tends to occur after Christmas. When influenza is known to be circulating widely in the community, the predictive value of clinical diagnosis is markedly improved. In England, influenza surveillance data can be readily accessed online at the Health Protection Agency website (www.hpa.org.uk). However it should also be recognized that influenza infections occur year round, and out-of-season activity is not infrequently detected in schools and residential homes for the elderly (even if most residents have been vaccinated).

Under circumstances where the clinician has a high degree of suspicion of influenza but this is outside of a known period of community activity, and especially when a treatment decision needs to be made, it is appropriate in both primary and secondary care settings to take a combined nose/throat swab (2 x plain cotton swabs placed into the same container containing virus transport medium) and request rapid influenza diagnostics from an appropriate local laboratory. The same is true for suspected influenza in outbreak-prone settings such as boarding schools and residential homes or where an outbreak is already apparent; under the latter circumstances, the local Health Protection Unit should be contacted at the earliest possible opportunity for advice.

Influenza is usually a self-limiting disease of around 5 days duration, but a severe and sometimes fatal primary viral pneumonia is occasionally described. The latter is recognized clinically by an influenza-like illness which progresses rapidly (typically within 24–48 hours) to produce dyspnoea, hypoxia, and sometimes frank

> ### Box 7.2 Diagnosis of influenza
>
> - Utilize surveillance data as well as clinical judgement; predictive value of clinical diagnosis improves during periods of known community activity
> - Fever, cough and malaise + rapid onset are cardinal diagnostic features
> - Virological diagnosis is important outside known influenza periods and in outbreak situations; outbreaks in residential settings are well documented to occur out-of-season
> - Contact the local Health Protection Unit if an outbreak is suspected in a community setting, or the Infection Control Team in a hospital setting.

respiratory distress. In such patients, the most common abnormality on auscultation of the chest is bilateral crackles; and radiological investigation most often reveals perihilar or diffuse interstitial infiltrates. Progression to Acute Respiratory Distress Syndrome (ARDS) is not uncommon, nor is the need for oxygen supplementation and ventilatory support. Secondary bacterial pneumonia is far more commonly associated with seasonal influenza, but tends to appear longer (several days) after the initial onset of symptoms. However, distinguishing between viral and bacterial pneumonia is not reliable based purely on clinical or radiological grounds and patients in difficulty with an ILI should be rapidly investigated for viral and bacterial pathogens. The commonest secondary bacterial organisms described are *S. pneumoniae*, *S. aureus* and *H. influenzae*.

A range of other secondary complications may also occur including: acute bronchitis, otitis media (in children), myocarditis, pericarditis, and neurological sequelae (febrile convulsions and Reye's syndrome in children; encephalitis). Influenza is associated with more severe outcomes in: neonates and children <2 years; the elderly, especially those over 75 years; and persons with underlying co-morbidities (e.g. asthma, diabetes, COPD, cardiac failure) in whom the acute infection may destabilise the underlying condition. In these groups, hospitalisation is not uncommon. This emphasizes the need to treat such patients early with a neuraminidase inhibitor (standard adult dosage: oseltamivir (Tamiflu®) 75mg b.d. by mouth or zanamivir (Relenza®) 10mg b.d. by oral inhalation). In England, NHS use of these drugs in primary care is limited by the National Institute for Health and Clinical Excellence (NICE) to the elderly persons with underlying high-risk conditions (chronic pulmonary or cardiac disease, diabetes, renal dysfunction and immune suppression – see www.nice.org.uk); however it remains legal for GPs to prescribe outside of these risk groups by private prescription (including to their own patients). In all cases where influenza is suspected and treatment with an antiviral is recommended by NICE, this should not be deferred pending the results of virological testing, since early instigation of therapy improves outcomes. NICE guidance does not apply in hospitals where it would be reasonable to treat any patient with moderate or severe influenza (confirmed or suspected) regardless of underlying co-morbidities.

Neuraminidase inhibitors modestly reduce the time to resolution of symptoms by 1-2 days; but more importantly, further data suggest that the risk of hospital admission and complications may also be reduced. Newer data suggest that mortality in patients hospitalized due to seasonal influenza is reduced by antiviral treatment. Finally, emerging data from the 2009 A/H1N1 pandemic suggest that for confirmed cases of pandemic influenza, the risks of hospitalization and severe outcome were both reduced by early antiviral treatment. For most patients, oseltamivir is probably the drug of choice, being relatively easy to administer and having a wider licensed age range than zanamivir. However zanamivir may be preferred in pregnancy due to its low bio-availability, and in severe renal insufficiency; it would also be the drug of choice in situations where resistance to oseltamivir was suspected or identified, e.g. an A/H1N1 virus carrying the H275Y mutation. Both drugs are licensed to be started within 48 hours of symptom onset, because beyond this point the effect on symptom reduction is marginal; and both are licensed for 5 days therapy. However, hospital practitioners confronted with a severely ill patient with proven influenza, suggestive of active virus replication, or GPs attending a patient in the community who is extremely unwell with an influenza-like illness, should not hesitate to start therapy >48 hours after symptom onset, nor to continue therapy for >5 days. Full prescribing information for both drugs can be obtained at www.medicines.org.uk.

Both oseltamivir and zanamivir are also licensed for prophylactic use, either as post-exposure prophylaxis (10 days therapy) or as longer term pre-exposure prophylaxis (up to 42 days). NICE guidance specifically allows for post-exposure use in the community where a high-risk individual, unprotected by vaccine, has been exposed to influenza; and use in the control of outbreaks. The latter is a highly specialized application, best supervised by health protection or hospital infection control specialists. However it should be stressed that primary care professionals and ward staff are usually best placed to raise the alarm about outbreaks of influenza in community residential settings and in hospital, where the emphasis should be on rapid response because mortality may be considerable among the institutionalised elderly and in specialist units treating patients with profound immune suppression.

7.3 **Influenza vaccines**

Influenza is currently the only respiratory virus infection which is vaccine preventable. Licensed human influenza vaccines have been available since 1945, following successful trials in the US military. They are now used extensively across the globe to prevent complications and death in patients at high-risk; and their safety record is excellent. In general, for seasonal influenza, the groups targeted for vaccination are the elderly (≥65 years), and patients of any age (vaccines are licensed from 6 months upwards) with underlying high-risk conditions. Typically these include: chronic pulmonary or cardiovascular conditions; diabetes mellitus; renal disease; and conditions or therapies producing immunosupression. In recent years, far greater attention has been focussed on the unrecognized burden of influenza in children and a few countries now offer vaccination to young children irrespective of underlying illnesses. It seems likely (and indeed sensible) that many countries will extend their recommendations to include young children over the next few years.

Prior to the influenza A/H1N1 pandemic in 2009, only a handful of countries offered influenza vaccine during pregnancy even though the risk to pregnant women was well-documented during the pandemics of the 20th century. However the 2009 pandemic has further highlighted the risks of influenza in pregnancy, and almost all countries with access to A/H1N1 pandemic vaccines have targeted pregnant women as a very high priority. Again, it seems likely (and sensible) that many countries will routinely target pregnant women for seasonal vaccination in the post-pandemic period. Solid data now exist demonstrating that maternal vaccination during pregnancy confers protection to the new born infant at a time when the baby is especially vulnerable to influenza and too young to receive licensed vaccines.

Most modern influenza seasonal vaccines are killed vaccines containing influenza surface antigens or split virus. In the majority of cases, production is still based on virus culture in embryonated hens' eggs. The biggest practical difficulty relates to the need for re-vaccination at the beginning of every winter season, because as the wild influenza viruses in circulation mutate over time, so too must the vaccine be altered to maintain its protective efficacy. In most but not all years, the match between vaccine and wild antigens is usually good. Modern seasonal vaccines are considered to be safe and effective. Numerous studies demonstrate reductions in mortality and hospitalization in elderly and high-risk patients that amount to solid public health benefits when applied at population level. Nevertheless, it is recognized that influenza vaccines are not as immunogenic in children and the elderly as in working age adults, and that there is therefore room for improvement. The global response to a possible influenza pandemic derived from A/H5N1 avian influenza, and the recent A/H1N1 pandemic are two events which have provided the stimulus for the successful development and deployment of new vaccines which either contain adjuvants, or are whole virus products, based on cell-culture. These two technologies may well be incorporated into future seasonal influenza vaccines to improve immunogenicity and/or extend the degree of cross-protection between strains.

7.4 **RSV management**

RSV is the commonest cause of respiratory virus infection in young children <2 years of age (mainly causing acute bronchiolitis) and is responsible for a very large number of annual hospital admissions in young children, mainly in winter. Nosocomial outbreaks on paediatric wards are also well documented, emphasising the need for well-enforced droplet and contact infection control precautions in this setting. Treatment of RSV is mainly supportive. Aerosolized ribavirin (Virazole®) is the only specific treatment available but is complex to administer and not that effective. Therefore it is important that children who are at high risk of hospitalisation and death due to RSV are identified and offered immunoprophylaxis with the recombinant human monoclonal antibody palivizumab (Synagis®), as no vaccine is yet available.

Box 7.3 UK recommendations for palivizumab immunoprophylaxis, 2009

- Children who have chronic lung disease (oxygen dependency for at least 28 days from birth) who have specific risk factors:
  - *infants under 3 months old at the start of the RSV season who were born at 30 weeks gestational age or less*
  - *infants under 6 months old at the start of the RSV season who were born at 26 weeks gestational age or less.*
- Children who have chronic lung disease (in other words oxygen dependency for at least 28 days from birth), and who also have a sibling in day care or school including:
  - *infants under 3 months old at the start of the RSV season who were born at 35 weeks gestational age or less*
  - *infants under 6 months old at the start of the RSV season who born at 30 weeks gestational age or less*
  - *infants under 9 months old at the start of the RSV season who born at 26 weeks gestational age or less.*
- Infants who have haemodynamically significant, acyanotic congenital heart disease and are less than 6 months old.
- Children who have severe combined immunodeficiency syndrome (SCID) until immune reconstituted.

Palivizumab is given by monthly intramuscular injection (usually up to 5 doses per winter season) and should be undertaken under specialist guidance. Therapy should be commenced before the start of the RSV season. Thankfully the timing of RSV activity in the UK is much more consistent than is the case for influenza and tends to begin during week 43 each autumn (mid-October), lasting until around week 11 (mid-March).

RSV is also a source of substantial morbidity and mortality in adults, especially the elderly. Transmission from children to grand-parents is strongly suspected, as diagnoses of acute bronchitis consistently peak before Christmas in children, but after New Year in the elderly. Recognition of the burden of illness in adults, espe-cially the elderly, has been somewhat slower to materialise than for children; but excess admissions and excess mortality in those over 65 years due to RSV activity (and previously wrongly attributed to influenza) have now been clearly defined. The contribution of RSV to serious adult respiratory infection, in addition to its more promi-nent burden in children, further emphasises the pressing need for safe and effective vaccines against this important virus.

Further reading

Cowling B.J., Chan K.H., Fang V.J., *et al.* (2010) Comparative epidemiology of pandemic and seasonal influenza A in households. *N Engl J Med* **362**(23): 2175–84.

Fleming D.M., Elliot A.J., Nguyen-Van-Tam J.S., Watson J.M., Wise R. (2005) A Winter's Tale. Coming to terms with winter respiratory illnesses. London: Health Protection Agency, http://www.hpa.org.uk/HPA/Publications/InfectiousDiseases/RespiratoryDiseases (accessed, October 2009)

Goddard N.L., Cooke M.C., Gupta R.K., Nguyen-Van-Tam J.S. (2007) Timing of monoclonal antibody for seasonal RSV prophylaxis in the United Kingdom. *Epidemiol Infect* **135**(1): 159–62.

Hessel L. Vaccines. In: Van-Tam, J., Sellwood, C. (eds). *Introduction to Pandemic Influenza*. Wallingford: CAB International: pp. 118–35.

Jain S., Kamimoto L., Bramley A.M., *et al.* (2009) Hospitalized patients with 2009 H1N1 influenza in the United States, April-June 2009. *N Engl J Med* **361**(20): 1935–44.

McGeer A., Green K.A., Plevneshi A., Shigayeva A., Siddiqi N., Raboud J., Low, D.E. (2007) Toronto Invasive Bacterial Diseases Network. Antiviral therapy and outcomes of influenza requiring hospitalization in Ontario, Canada. *Clin Infect Dis* **45**(12): 1568–75.

National Institute for Health and Clinical Excellence (2009) Amantadine, oseltamivir and zanamivir for the treatment of influenza. Review of NICE technology appraisal guidance 58. http://guidance.nice.org.uk/TA168/Guidance/pdf/English (accessed, October 2009).

Nguyen-Van-Tam J.S., Openshaw P.J., Hashim A., *et al.* Influenza Clinical Information Network (FLU-CIN). (2010) Risk factors for hospitalisation and poor outcome with pandemic A/H1N1 influenza: United Kingdom first wave (May-September 2009). *Thorax* **65**(7): 645–51.

Nicholson K.G., McNally T., Silverman M., Simons P., Stockton J.D., Zambon M.C. (2006) Rates of hospitalisation for influenza, respiratory syncytial virus and human metapneumovirus among infants and young children. *Vaccine* **24**(1): 102–8.

Puleston R.L., Bugg G., Hoschler K., *et al.* (2010) Observational study to investigate vertically acquired passive immunity in babies of mothers vaccinated against H1N1v during pregnancy. *Health Technol Assess* **14**(55): 1–82.

Samransamruajkit R., Hiranrat T., Chieochansin T., Sritippayawan S., Deerojanawong J., Prappha N., Poovorawan Y. (2008) Prevalence, clinical presentations and complicatiosns among hospitalized children with influenza pneumonia. *Jpn J Infect Dis* **61**(6): 446–9.

Van Kerkhove M.D., Vandemaele K.A., Shinde V., *et al.* on behalf of the WHO Working Group for Risk Factors for Severe H1N1pdm Infection. (2011) Risk Factors for Severe Outcomes following 2009 Influenza A (H1N1) Infection: A Global Pooled Analysis. *PLoS Med* **8**(7): e1001053.

Viboud C., Miller M., Olson D. (2010) Preliminary Estimates of Mortality and Years of Life Lost Associated with the 2009 A/H1N1 Pandemic in the US and Comparison with Past Influenza Seasons. *PLoS Curr* **20**: RRN1153.

Writing Committee of the WHO Consultation on Clinical Aspects of Pandemic (H1N1) Influenza (2009), Bautista E., Chotpitayasunondh T., Gao Z., *et al.* (2010) Clinical aspects of pandemic 2009 influenza A (H1N1) virus infection. N Engl J Med. 2010 May 6;362(18):1708–19. Review. *N Engl J Med* **362**(21): 2039.

Chapter 8

Pneumococcal respiratory disease and vaccines

Thomas Bewick and Wei Shen Lim

> **Key points**
> - *Streptococcus pneumoniae* is the predominant bacterial pathogen implicated in all lower respiratory tract infections
> - The organism's pathogenicity is to a large extent due to its polysaccharide capsule, which also enables classification into different serotypes/serogroups
> - Risk factors associated with pneumococcal pneumonia include HIV infection, defects in humoral immunity, asplenia, diabetes mellitus, cancer, high alcohol intake, smoking and the extremes of age
> - Pneumococcal urinary antigen detection kits enable a rapid and accurate diagnosis of pneumococcal infection
> - Adult pneumococcal vaccination with **polysaccharide** vaccine does not reduce the incidence of community-acquired pneumonia, but may attenuate its severity
> - Childhood pneumococcal vaccination with **conjugate** vaccine is highly effective at reducing all pneumococcal disease in children and may also provide beneficial effects in unvaccinated children and adults as a result of herd protection

8.1 Introduction

Streptococcus pneumoniae (the 'pneumococcus') is a Gram positive diplococcus responsible for the majority of bacterial respiratory infections worldwide. It is the principle cause of community-acquired pneumonia (CAP), otitis media (OM), and non-pneumonic lower respiratory tract infection (LRTI) (Table 8.1). It is also the cause of invasive disease such as bacterial meningitis (especially in the very young and old), septicaemia, and endocarditis.

Table 8.1 The proportion of disease thought to be attributable to *S. pneumoniae* in different medical conditions

Medical condition	Proportion of disease caused by *S. pneumoniae*
All lower respiratory tract infections (LRTIs)	17–30%
Non-pneumonic LRTI	8–14%
Community acquired pneumonia	> 50%
Otitis media	28–55%

8.2 **From carriage to infection**

8.2.1 **Nasopharyngeal carriage**

Streptococcus pneumoniae can normally be found as part of the nasopharyngeal mucous membrane microflora. Such colonization usually does not result in any symptoms. However, carriers act as a reservoir for transmission to others and it is generally thought that pneumococci in the nasopharynx are the source of pneumococcal infection in the same individual. The prevalence of pneumococcal nasopharyngeal carriage is strongly associated with the age and contact with pneumococcal carriers. In developing countries, newborns may become colonised with pneumococci within days following birth. Nasopharyngeal carriage rates in young children (especially infants) range between 50% to 90%. Beyond 10 years of age, carriage rates drop below 10%. In affluent countries, pneumococcal colonisation is often delayed till a few months after birth and prevalence rates at 2 years of age are around 40% to 50% and start to drop by age 5 years of age. From the few data available, carriage rates in the elderly are thought to be very low. Transmission from person to person is via contact with respiratory secretions from carriers.

8.2.2 **Pathogenesis**

Streptococcus pneumoniae causes disease when it encounters an area of the body where it is not a commensal organism, such as the alveolus or middle ear. The mechanism of transition from commensal to pathogen is not fully understood. Conditions such as immune suppression or co-existent viral infection appear to promote this transition. In the lungs, resident alveolar macrophages can phagocytose low levels of bacteria, but failure to adequately clear the bacteria results in activation of the other arms of the host innate immune response, resulting in cytokine release, activation of the complement cascade, and attraction of neutrophils to the site of infection. Subsequently bacteria may enter the blood stream and seed to other sites such as the heart valves, meninges or joints.

The pneumococcus has a polysaccharide-containing capsule surrounding the cell wall, which helps to protect the bacterium from immunological attack, particularly by preventing opsonisation by immunoglobulins and complement and subsequent phagocytosis. Capsular variation is responsible for different patterns of disease and virulence, and allows characterization of *S. pneumoniae* into over 90 serotypes/serogroups. The spleen contains macrophages that are key to removing opsonized pneumococci; hence asplenic patients are at particular risk of pneumococcal disease. Other recognized risk factors associated with pneumococcal pneumonia include HIV infection, abnormal humoural immunity (defects in complement or immunoglobulin), diabetes mellitus, cancer, high alcohol intake, smoking and the extremes of age.

8.2.3 Clinical disease

Characteristic features of pneumococcal pneumonia that have been described include an abrupt onset of illness, pleuritic chest pain, and rust-coloured or blood-tinged sputum. However, these features are not specific for pneumococcal infection and it is generally acknowledged that pneumococcal lower respiratory tract infections cannot be reliably distinguished clinically from similar infections caused by other respiratory pathogens. Importantly, the clinical presentation of pneumococcal pneumonia caused by penicillin-sensitive and resistant strains does not appear to differ significantly. In contrast, some differences according to serotype have been described. For instance, serotype 1 has been associated with childhood pneumoccoal empyema in the United States and United Kingdom.

Occasionally, patients present with only extra-pulmonary symptoms, such as meningitis, severe sepsis or endocarditis. Rarer manifestations of pneumococcal disease include pericarditis and peritonitis. Austrian's triad refers to the concurrence of bacteremic pneumococcal pneumonia, meningitis, and endocarditis; a rare and virulent presentation of invasive pneumococcal disease named after Dr Robert Austrian—a major figure in pneumococcal research who described the syndrome. Patients with HIV have a higher rate of invasive disease compared to immunocompetent individuals.

8.3 Diagnosis

Invasive pneumococcal disease (IPD) may be detected by blood culture. However, this test is insensitive as a means of detection of pneumococcal infections; in routine practice, it is positive in only about 5% of all cases of CAP. Sputum culture and Gram stain are useful when an adequate sputum sample is obtained for analysis (ideally <10 epithelial cells and >25 white blood cells per low-power field magnification, x 10). Unfortunately, a substantial proportion of patients with lower respiratory tract infection either do not cough up sputum, or are unable to produce adequate samples. In addition, prior antibiotic use greatly reduces the diagnostic rate. Even a single oral dose of penicillin can render subsequent blood and sputum cultures negative.

A diagnostic test for *S. pneumoniae* with reasonable sensitivity (65–75%) and good specificity (94–100%) is an immunochromatographic assay which detects fragments of pneumococcal capsular polysaccharide. Although this assay has primarily been validated on urine samples, it has also been used successfully on pleural fluid. When applied to patients with CAP, it can increase the proportion of patients in whom a diagnosis of pneumococcal infection is made (over and above sputum and blood cultures) by >25%. A further advantage is that unlike other microbiological methods that depend on bacterial culture, antigen detection is less affected by prior antibiotic use. The assay is commercially marketed as a 'bedside' diagnostic kit with results obtainable in 15 minutes.

8.4 **Pneumococcal polysaccharide vaccine**

Pneumococcal vaccines work by inducing protective antibody responses to the capsular polysaccharide antigens, and are typically defined by the number of different serotypes covered (their 'valency'). The first pneumococcal vaccine introduced in 1977 for adults was 14-valent. This was replaced by a 23-valent polysaccharide vaccine (PPV-23; Pneumovax®) which has been used in the UK since 1983. The 23 capsular polysaccharide components of PPV represent the commonest pneumococcal serotypes which together account for 88% of worldwide invasive pneumococcal disease in adults. Vaccine coverage includes those serotypes implicated in most invasive disease or in antibiotic resistance (Table 8.2). The breadth of protection is further improved by cross-reactivity of some serotypes contained within the vaccine with others that are not (for example, 6A and 6B). This increases vaccine coverage by an additional 8%.

8.4.1 **Target groups**

In many countries, vaccination with PPV-23 is offered to younger adults who are at-risk of pneumococcal disease (Box 8.1) and to older adults (≥65 years of age) without specific risk factors. It is not appropriate for use in children aged less than 2 years due to their relatively immature immune system. In the immunocompetent adult, the vaccine only needs to be given once and protection should last at least 5 years. In some immunocompromised adults a second dose may be given 5 years after the initial vaccination.

Box 8.1 Definition of at-risk groups for whom pneumococcal vaccines are recommended. Note that there is some variation between countries
Group or condition
Age >65 years or <2 years
Asthma
Chronic obstructive pulmonary disease
Chronic kidney disease
Immunosuppressed state / HIV
Hyposplenism
Congestive cardiac failure
Chronic liver disease
Diabetes
Adult smokers (in the US)

8.4.2 **Efficacy**

Polysaccharides, as contained in PPV-23, are poorly immunogenic when compared with proteins, and only induce a T cell-independent response. Between 75% and 85% of healthy adults will mount a good antibody response to vaccination. However, the elderly, those with severe co-morbidity, patients with HIV and patients who are functionally hyposplenic produce far lower responses. In addition, the relationship between antibody levels and protection from IPD is not certain. PPV-23 has not been conclusively shown to prevent CAP, either on an outpatient basis or as measured by admissions to hospital, and has not been shown to reduce mortality from CAP. Nevertheless, it has an efficacy of between 30% and 45% in reducing the incidence of invasive pneumococcal disease. Some data also suggest that PPV-23 vaccinated individuals who develop CAP have less severe disease as measured by reduced admission rates to critical care.

8.4.3 **HIV infection**

The immune responses generated by PPV-23 are attenuated in the HIV-infected population, especially in patients with lower CD4 cell counts. Patients on anti-retroviral therapy appear to gain more protection from vaccination although the response remains sub-optimal, even after re-vaccination. Current guidelines recommend the use of

PPV-23 in HIV-infected patients with CD4 counts of >200 cells/µl, and recommend consideration of the vaccine in those with CD4 counts <200 cells/µl, though the evidence for benefit is not certain.

8.4.4 Re-vaccination

Antibody levels fall after 5–10 years in the healthy adult, but it is not known whether vaccine efficacy decreases with time. As it induces a T cell-independent response, it is not possible to produce a 'booster' effect by administering a repeat vaccination. Re-vaccination results in lower antibody rises than following the first vaccination, and a higher rate of local side effects. Repeat vaccination may also reduce additional responses to antigen challenge ('hyporesponsiveness'). Consequently re-vaccination should never be offered within 3 years of first vaccination, and is usually only considered in later years in patients at high risk of pneumococcal disease.

Table 8.2 Pneumococcal vaccine serotype coverage. PPV; pneumococcal polysaccharide vaccine. PCV; pneumococcal conjugate vaccine

Vaccine	Serotypes covered
PPV-23	1, 2, 3, 4, 5, 6B, 7F, 8, 9N, 9V, 10A, 11A, 12F, 14, 15B, 17F, 18C, 19A, 19F, 20, 22F, 23F, 33F
PCV-7	4, 6B, 9V, 14, 18C, 19F, 23F
PCV-10	1, 4, 5, 6B, 7F, 9V, 14, 18C, 19F, 23F
PCV-13	1,3,4, 5, 6A, 6B, 7F, 9V, 14, 18C, 19A, 19F, 23F

8.5 Pneumococcal conjugate vaccine

Conjugate vaccines involve the combination (conjugation) of pneumococcal capsular polysaccharides with an immunogenic protein (e.g. derived from diphtheria). This provokes a T cell-dependent response, inducing immunological memory and therefore theoretically conferring greater protection. A 7-valent pneumococcal conjugate vaccine (PCV-7) was introduced to the childhood immunization schedule in the US in 2000 and to the UK in September 2006. In 2010, both countries switched to a 13-valent vaccine (PCV-13) which includes the original 7 serotypes in PCV-7 plus 6 additional serotypes. At least a further 24 countries offer PCV as part of a routine childhood immunization schedule. Most regimens comprise 3 vaccinations at 2, 4 and 13 months of age, taking advantage of the 'booster effect' that immunological memory confers. The 13-valent PCV offers coverage of the 13 serotypes representing the majority of childhood pneumococcal disease globally. (Table 8.3)

Table 8.3 Approximate proportions of IPD in children <5 years of age due to serotypes in PCV-13. (data from Johnson HL et al. Plos Med 2010 Oct 5;7(10). pii: e1000348.)	
Region	Childhood IPD due to PCV-13 serotypes (%)
Africa	76
Asia	74
Europe	88
Latin America and Caribbean	83
North America	88
Oceania	80
Global	75

These serotypes include those associated with the majority of pneumococcal penicillin resistance.

8.5.1 Efficacy and herd protection

PCV generates antibody responses in between 60% and 100% of infants vaccinated. In contrast to PPV, PCV has been shown to reduce the incidence not only of childhood invasive pneumococcal disease (90% reduction of vaccine-type), but also childhood CAP (25–37% reduction). PCV-7 also induces stronger IgA responses than PPV, accounting for a 6–7% reduction in otitis media.

Anti-pneumococcal IgA serves to reduce nasopharyngeal carriage of serotypes covered by the vaccine. This is thought to promote herd protection with consequent reduction in the burden of pneumococcal disease in non-vaccinated children and adults. For instance, childhood vaccination has been shown to reduce carriage within non-vaccinated adults in the same household, and since the introduction of childhood PCV vaccination in the US, rates of adult IPD have also fallen significantly.

8.6 Future vaccine developments

The 13-valent PCV is currently being evaluated for use in older adults, where it is hoped that the improved immunogenicity of PCV will enhance the prevention of IPD and CAP in this age group. Fifteen valent vaccines have also been developed to further extend serotype coverage. However, manufacturing difficulties limit the number of valencies that can be reasonably incorporated into a single vaccine.

As the use of PCVs increase, serotype replacement may occur as the prevalence of non-vaccine serotypes increase. Close monitoring of prevailing serotypes is therefore necessary.

Other vaccine developments involve targeting non-capsular protein-based antigens which would in theory provide protection against all pneumococcal serotypes, and the adjuvant stimulation of innate immune responses to improve host defences.

Further reading

Braido F., Bellotti M., Maria A., *et al.* (2008) The role of pneumococcal vaccine. *Pulm Pharmacol Ther* **21**: 608–15.

Grijalva C.G., Nuorti J.P., Arbogast P.G., Martin S.W., Edwards K.M., Griffin M.R. (2007) Decline in pneumonia admissions after routine childhood immunisation with pneumococcal conjugate vaccine in the USA: a time-series analysis. *Lancet* **369**(9568): 1179–86.

Huss A., Scott P., Stuck A.E., Trotter C., Egger M. (2009) Efficacy of pneumo-coccal vaccination in adults: a meta-analysis. *CMAJ* **180**(1): 48–58.

Johnson H.L., Deloria-Knoll M., Levine O.S., *et al.* (2010) Systemic evalua-tion of serotypes causing invasive pneumococcal disease among children under five: the pneumococcal global serotype project. *PLoS Med* **7**(10). pii:e1000348.

van der Poll T., Opal S.M. (2009) Pathogenesis, treatment and prevention of pneumococcal pneumonia. *Lancet* **374**: 1543–56.

Chapter 9

Legionnaires' disease

John Macfarlane

Key points

- Legionnaires' disease is an uncommon but important cause of pneumonia with a unique mode of spread
- Legionella infection tends to result in moderate or severe pneumonia sometimes complicated by respiratory and other organ failure and is associated with a 12% mortality overall
- Early diagnosis and management has been revolutionized with the availability of a rapid legionella urinary antigen test
- The legionella urinary antigen test should be requested on all patients presenting with severe pneumonia, and also for those whom legionella is suspected for epidemiological or other reasons
- A fluoroquinolone is the preferred antibiotic for proven legionella pneumonia
- Investigating the source of the infection is essential in preventing further cases.

9.1 Introduction and historical context

Legionnaires' disease is a relatively uncommon but important cause of pneumonia due to its unique mode of infection, potential severity of illness, significant morbidity and mortality, lack of response to penicillins and other β-lactam antibiotics, and the importance of identifying the source of infection to prevent further cases.

The name derives from the defining outbreak of a previously unrecognized acute severe pneumonia that affected former soldiers, or Legionnaires, who had recently attended a convention at the Bellevue Stratford Hotel in Philadelphia, Pennsylvania in 1976. It was several months before a newly identified organism, *Legionella pneumophila* was discovered to have been the cause of the pneumonia which affected 221 American Legionnaires, of whom

34 died. Since then it has been recognized as a cause of explosive outbreaks of illness as well as causing isolated single cases or small clusters of illness worldwide. The term 'legionellosis' is used to describe the clinical illness caused by legionella infection, which can present either as Legionnaires' disease (pneumonia) or Pontiac fever (a non-pneumonic short-lived influenza-like illness).

The Legionellaceae are Gram-negative bacilli with distinctive cell walls. Of the 50 or so recognized legionella species, *L. pneumophila* serogroup 1 is responsible for most cases in North America and Europe and accounts for over 80% in the UK. Other serogroups or species can cause infection in immunocompromised patients or be associated with certain geographical areas. For example, *L. long-beachae* accounts for about half of cases of Legionnaires' disease in Australia and New Zealand, and is also found in parts of SE Asia. This species is unusual, being soil dwelling, and transmission has been linked to gardening and the use of moist potting composts.

9.2 Mode of infection and pathology

Pathogenesis is influenced by the fact that legionellae are intracellular pathogens, both in natural and manmade water systems and also in the human lung where they can exist relatively protected from external influences. They reach the lung following inhalation of infected water aerosols. There, they are taken up by and multiply within alveolar macrophages by preventing normal cellular bacterial killing. The lungs show a severe inflammatory response, principally involving mononuclear cells and fibrin. Unlike other causes of bacterial pneumonia, blood stream spread of the organism is unusual and the lungs remain the principal organ affected, except in severely immunocompromised patients. Case to case transmission does not occur and isolation of a case is unnecessary.

Legionellae are ubiquitous in natural water habitats and man made water systems. Legionellae thrive at temperatures of 25°C to 45°C, and are inhibited and then killed as temperatures are raised above 55°C. In water systems, warmth, impurities, sludge, and water stagnation can all contribute to rapid multiplication. Once colonized, eradication is difficult as the legionellae live within amoebae in the biofilm. Wet cooling towers are an important cause of large outbreaks of legionellosis. Wet towers depend on the cooling effect of recycled water falling down over and evaporating on water pipes in the towers. The resultant drift of legionella-containing water aerosols can travel considerable distances from such evaporative cooling towers often positioned on roofs of large buildings, and infect people over wide areas downwind. Within buildings, both cold and hot water pipe work can become easily colonized where a range of appliances can facilitate the dissemination of contaminated aerosols.

Most commonly, showers are implicated but other well recognized sources include decorative fountains, whirlpool spas (jacuzzis), mist-cooled cabinets, automatic car washes, and sprays used to cool grinding and drilling tools in factories. Some outbreaks have been linked to airborne exposure to moist potting compost (particularly *L. longbeachae*) and earth particles. Increasingly cases have been linked to domestic water. In the UK, about half of cases reported are related to travel, mostly abroad, about half are sporadic and community acquired, and only about 5% nosocomial. Recent stays in hotels, hospitals or visits to large buildings and leisure facilities may thus provide a clue to the possibility of Legionnaires' disease in patient presenting with pneumonia. However the diverse sources of infection means that legionella infection may not initially be considered when taking a history from a new patient with pneumonia.

Legionellosis is seasonal being commoner in the summer and autumn partly due to increased exposure to water systems such as showers and air conditioning and also travel to holiday hotels.

Following the lead from most of Europe, legionellosis is now notifiable in England and Wales. However the majority of UK laboratories have reported cases to central databases for many years. Since 1980, over 6,500 cases have been documented in England and Wales and over 8,300 reported to the European Working Group on Legionella Infections in the last two decades.

However legionella infection causes only around 2–5% of cases of sporadic community acquired pneumonia in the UK, although there is geographical variation. Clusters and outbreaks also occur—the last large outbreak in the UK affected 180 people with seven deaths in August 2002 in the coastal town of Barrow in North West England. Because legionella infection has a tendency to cause moderate or severe illness, hospital admission is often needed, usually within less than a week of symptom onset, and mild illness in the community is less usual than with pneumococcal or mycoplasma pneumonia. In about a fifth of hospitalized cases, critical care management is required for ventilatory and other organ failure. Legionella pneumonia is the second commonest cause (after pneumococcal pneumonia) of community acquired pneumonia requiring admission to the intensive care unit. Men are three times more frequently affected than woman and infection in childhood and in the elderly is less usual, with most patients being in the 40–70 year old range with a median of 59 years. Those at risk include cigarette smokers, alcoholics, those with reasons for immunosuppression or receiving corticosteroids, chronic illness, and diabetes. The incubation period is taken as 2–10 days, with a median of just under 7 days, and it is rare to be more than 14 days. This knowledge is important both for the clinician considering the diagnosis and the public health protection specialist considering the source.

9.3 Clinical features

There are no unique clinical or laboratory features of Legionnaires' disease that can allow a confident early clinical diagnosis and most cases present as an acute community acquired pneumonia of unknown cause.

However some patients show a collection of clinical features that should alert the clinician to the possibility of legionellosis (Box 9.1).

Clues on initial investigations may include a total white cell count only modestly raised to less than 15,000 per litre, hyponatraemia, abnormalities of liver function tests, raised muscle enzymes and a very high C-reactive protein. Blood and sputum cultures will reveal no predominant pathogen on routine testing and sputum Gram stain few pus cells. The chest radiograph usually shows homogeneous shadowing and characteristically the consolidation can spread quickly to the same or opposite lung, even if appropriate antibiotics have been started. Radiographic recovery can take many weeks in some survivors and some patients are left with linear lines suggestive of small areas of fibrosis or atelectasis.

Box 9.1 The presence of several of these clinical features should alert the clinician to the possibility of Legionnaires' disease

- Relevant epidemiological clues
- A short history of less than a week, with progressive moderate or severe pneumonia
- Relative paucity of respiratory symptoms. Productive cough, haemoptysis, upper respiratory tract symptoms and pleural pain seem *less* common compared with pneumococcal pneumonia
- Non-respiratory symptoms such as increasing headache, confusion, abnormal behaviour and diarrhoea can dominate the clinical picture.
- High fevers, sweating and rigors
- Multi-system features with abnormal investigations (see text)
- Non-response to β-lactam antibiotics such as penicillin.

9.4 Diagnosis

The diagnosis and consequently the early management of Legionnaires' disease has been revolutionized over the last decade due to the increasingly widespread availability of legionella urinary antigen detection systems. In the past, diagnosis often relied on follow up serology, or identifying the organism by stain or culture in respiratory samples, sometimes obtained by invasive techniques. Urine antigen testing is now the mainstay of diagnosis, with a specificity and sensitivity of 90% for the best test systems. The test is usually positive at an early stage of infection and hence can guide early appropriate antibiotic therapy and source investigation. However an initial negative urine antigen test does not exclude the diagnosis, and further urine should be sent for repeat testing if clinically indicated, together with respiratory samples for legionella culture. Serology to detect an antibody response to legionellae can still be of value for making a late diagnosis by comparing acute and convalescent samples and demonstrating a fourfold or greater rise in antibody titre. The urine antigen test only reliably detects *Legionella pneumophila serogroup 1* infection (by far the commonest cause of community acquired legionella pneumonia in most countries) and this drawback must be remembered when investigating an immunocompromised patient or a nosocomial case who on occasions may be infected by other legionella species.

Even when the diagnosis of Legionnaires' disease has been confirmed by urinary antigen detection in a patient with pneumonia, it is still important to send respiratory secretions, such as sputum for specific legionella culture. This can be particularly helpful in matching the specific legionella bacteria subspecies and strain causing that clinical illness to cultures from environmental water sources, by monoclonal antibody subgrouping or by molecular typing, and hence identify the exact source of infection and prevent further cases.

It is recommended that urine should be sent for legionella bacterial antigen detection and respiratory secretions, such as sputum, sent for legionella culture from all patients with severe pneumonia and also from those with clinical or epidemiological pointers to Legionnaires' disease.

9.5 **Management**

Recommending an evidence based optimal antibiotic policy for Legionnaires' disease is difficult because there are no controlled prospective clinical trial data available. However laboratory studies and clinical experience in the form of case reports and observational studies lead to the recommendation that fluoroquinolones are the antibiotic of choice for proven Legionnaires' disease with most data being available for levofloxacin in both the intravenous and oral formulation. Alternative choices, if fluoroquinolones are contraindicated, include a macrolide such as clarithromycin (or erythromycin or azithromycin), and also tetracyclines and rifampicin (Box 9.2). Duration of antibiotics is similar as for other causes of community acquired pneumonia and is largely a matter of clinical judgement or habit. Seven to 10 days is a typical duration for uncomplicated cases.

For severe or life threatening pneumonia, most clinicians would consider adding an additional antibiotic, such as clarithromycin, to the fluoroquinolone therapy for the first few days. Clinicians should be alert to potential cardiac rhythm disturbances when using combined quinolones and macrolides. Rifampicin has been a popular alternative additional choice, but it acts as an enzyme inducer and can interact with other drug actions, and also cause hyperbilirubinaemia, which resolves on stopping the drug.

By contrast the self-limiting non-pneumonic influenza-like form of legionellosis called Pontiac fever resolves without the need for any antibiotics. Typically it causes illness 1 to 2 days after exposure and has a very high attack rate. The pathogenesis is not understood, but may possibly be a hypersensitivity response.

Box 9.2 Management of a case of Legionnaires' disease

Antibiotic management
- Use a fluoroquinolone as the preferred antibiotic
- Consider a macrolide such as clarithromycin (or erythromycin or azithromycin) as an alternative choice
- Consider combination antibiotics for the first few days in severe or life threatening Legionnaires' disease, but be alert to the possibility of drug interactions (see text)
- Use clinical judgement to dictate duration of antibiotic therapy.

General management
- Monitor and review regularly
- Be alert to the possibility of progressive respiratory failure and other organ failure
- Consider critical care review if condition worsening
- Manage oxygenation, hydration and nutrition
- Send off respiratory samples such as sputum specifically for legionella culture, to aid source identification.

Other specific issues
- Facilitate investigations by the local Public Health Specialist into potential source (in the UK, confirm with your Microbiology Department that the local Health Protection Unit has been informed promptly)
- Provide information, support and understanding to the patient and their relatives when telling them about the diagnosis.

The correct general management of the patient is also crucial with careful monitoring for clinical deterioration, particularly in the form of progressive respiratory failure requiring critical care input or mechanical ventilation. Appropriate oxygenation, hydration and nutrition are important. In the UK, all cases of Legionnaires' disease should be reported immediately to the local Health Protection Unit so that investigations can get under way to identify the potential source of the infection and prevent further cases. This will often involve a Public Health Specialist interviewing the patient or their relatives regarding movements in the previous 14 days. This and the ongoing public and media concern with Legionnaires' disease as a 'mysterious killer bug', together with the potential that the infection may have been caused by someone else's negligence regarding water system maintenance often means that the patient and their relatives require extra information, support and understanding from their clinical team.

9.6 **Prognosis and complications**

Although the early diagnosis and management of Legionnaires' disease has been revolutionized by the use of urine antigen testing, the mortality still remains around 12% with the outcome being adversely influenced by delay in the diagnosis or delay in the use of appropriate antibiotics and critical care. The most important early complication is acute respiratory failure. Up to 20% of cases require mechanical ventilation in some series. Other organ failure (cardiac and renal) also occurs. Anecdotally, recovery appears slower than with other types of bacterial pneumonia and it is not unusual for survivors to be troubled by debility, memory and concentration impairment, tiredness, muscle weakness, and various psychological sequelae for weeks or months after hospital discharge.

Some patients may get involved in civil litigation where it has been shown that a person or organization (such as a hotel or holiday company) negligently exposed the person to infected water aerosols. There is now a raft of legislation regarding the prevention and control of legionellae in buildings and water systems. On occasions, action may be taken through the criminal courts by the legislatory authorities where breaches of health and safety legislation have contributed to deaths from Legionnaires' disease.

9.7 **Prevention**

This is important at several levels. The key to prevention is the correct design and maintenance of man-made water systems and there is now widespread advice, schedules, and legislation to cover all aspects of legionella control in engineering practice. From the clinician's point of view, the most important aspect of prevention is first making a diagnosis of legionellosis and then ensuring this triggers a prompt investigation, identification and control of the possible source of infection to prevent further cases.

Further reading

Blazquez Garrido R.M., Parra F.J.E., Frances L.A. *et al.* (2005) Antimicrobial chemotherapy for legionnaires' disease: Levofloxacin versus Macrolides. *Clinical Infectious Diseases* **40**: 800–6.

British Thoracic Society (2009) Guidelines of the management of community acquired pneumonia in adults. *Thorax*, **64**: iii1–iii55.

Cunha B.A. (1998) Clinical features of legionnaires' disease. *Seminars in Respiratory Infections* **13**: 116–27.

Den Boer J.W., Nijhof J., Friesema I. (2006) Risk factors for sporadic community acquired Legionnaires' disease. A 3 year national case-controlled study. *Public Health* **120**: 566–71.

Health and Safety Commission (2000). *Legionnaires' Disease: the control of legionella bacteria in water systems Approved code of practice and guidance L8* HSE Books, Sudbury, Suffolk, UK.

Lee J.V., Joseph C. (2002) Guidelines for investigating single cases of legionnaires' disease. *Communicable Disease and Public Health* **5**: 157–62.

Lettinga K.D., Verbon A., Weverling G.J. *et al.* (2002) Legionnaires' disease at a Dutch flower show: prognostic factors and impact of therapy. *Emerging Infectious Diseases* **8**: 1448–54.

Phares C.R., Wangroongsarb P., Chantra S., *et al.* (2007) Epidemiology of severe pneumonia caused by Legionella longbeachae, Mycoplasma pneumoniae and Chlamydia pneumoniae: 1 year population based surveillance for severe pneumonia in Thailand. *Clinical Infectius Disease* **45**: 147–155.

Pedro-Botet, L. and Yu V.L. (2006) Legionella: macrolides or quinolones? *Clin Microbiol Infect* **12**(3): 25–30.

Woodhead M.A., Macfarlane J.T. (1985) The protean manifestations of Legionnaires' disease. *Journal of the Royal College Physicians (London)* **19**: 224–30.

Woodhead M.A., Macfarlane J.T. (1987) Comparative clinical and laboratory features of legionella with pneumococcal and mycoplasma pneumonias. *B J Dis Chest* **81**: 133–9.

Chapter 10

Less common and tropical respiratory tract infections

Wei Shen Lim

> ### Key points
>
> - Pulmonary actinomycosis has a world-wide distribution and may resemble lung cancer or tuberculosis
> - Tuberculosis may present as an acute pneumonia, especially in countries with high rates of tuberculosis
> - In countries where *Burkholderia pseudomallaei* ('melioidosis') is endemic, it is a common cause of severe community acquired pneumonia (CAP) that is not always covered by initial empirical antibiotics recommended for CAP in non-endemic areas
> - Most pneumonias associated with malaria are secondary bacterial pneumonias
> - A dry cough and non-specific chest x-ray changes are common in acute schistosomiasis.

101

10.1 Pulmonary actinomycosis

Actinomycosis has a world-wide distribution and may affect any age group, most commonly middle-aged men. Infection in children is uncommon. It is traditionally classified according to the region of involvement, namely cervicofacial, pulmonary, and abdomino-pelvic actinomycosis. Pulmonary infections are thought to occur as a result of aspiration of material infected with *Actinomyces sp.* facultative anaerobic Gram-positive bacteria that are normally found in the human oropharynx, especially in persons with poor dentition or poor oral hygiene. Alternatively, pulmonary involvement may be the result of direct spread from cervicofacial or abdominal infections. The infection does not respect anatomical boundaries and may spread from the lungs through the pleura and present as a chest wall mass (see Figure 10.1).

Fig 10.1 a Actinomycosis presenting as a chest wall mass

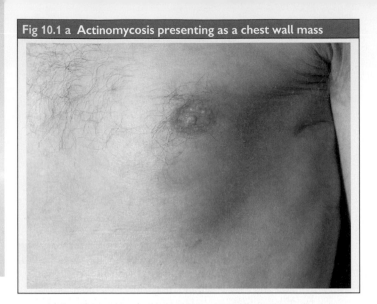

Fig 10.1 b Corresponding CT thorax of actinomycosis presenting as a chest wall mass

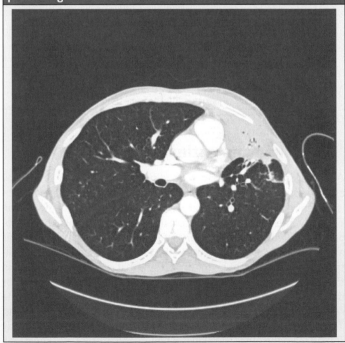

Patients with severe chronic lung disease are at higher risk of infection. The higher prevalence of alcoholism in patients with actinomycosis may be related to their risk of aspiration. Unusually, actinomycosis does not appear to be any commoner in patients with HIV or AIDS.

The commonest presentation is as a chronic debilitating illness associated with a shadow on chest radiography resembling lung cancer or tuberculosis. The most frequent symptoms reported are cough, sputum production, and chest pain. An acute fulminant presentation akin to acute pneumonia has been described in immunocompromised patients.

Other forms of pulmonary involvement include pleural empyema, pulmonary nodules, pulmonary cavities, miliary disease, and endobronchial obstruction. In all presentations, dissemination via the blood can result in multiple organ involvement.

10.1.1 **Diagnosis**

Due to the myriad possible presentations, a high index of suspicion is required to achieve an early diagnosis. Not uncommonly, the diagnosis is only made following histological examination of a surgically resected specimen.

The presence of sulpha granules in pus or in histological specimens is a characteristic finding. The granules consist of a basophilic core of micro-organisms surrounded by a radiating arrangement of eosinophilic poteinaceous material. Although sulpha granules are highly suggestive of actinomycosis, they are also occasionally seen in nocardiosis, chromomycosis, eumycetoma, and botryomycosis.

In most actinomycotic infections, apart from *Actinomyces sp.* (including *A israelii*—the commonest pathogen, *A naeslundii, A viscosus, A meyeri* and *Proprionibacterium proprionicum*), other organisms are also commonly found such as *Bacteroides, Fusobacterium, Capnocytophaga, Eikenella corrodens, Actinobacillus actinomycetemcomitans*, and *Enterobacteriaceae*. The role of these organisms in the pathogenesis of the disease is not certain.

10.1.2 **Treatment**

The treatment of choice is penicillin at high dose for a prolonged duration. In severe disease, initial treatment is with intravenous therapy for 2–6 weeks followed by oral therapy for 6–12 months to prevent relapse. In general, pulmonary actinomycosis appears to require longer treatment courses compared to other forms of actinomycosis. Tetracyclines have been used successfully as an alternative to penicillin. Surgical drainage of abscesses, or resection of infected material, may be required in addition to antibiotic therapy. Interestingly, the treatment of organisms other than *Actinomyces sp.* isolated in actinomycotic lesions, using antibiotics other than penicillin, has not been found to be a requirement for clinical cure.

10.2 **Community acquired pneumonia in the tropics**

There is often concern regarding the pathogens associated with pneumonia in patients returning from travels in Africa, the Indian subcontinent and the Far East, particularly when such travel has occurred within the tropics. Rigorous studies to determine the microbial aetiology of community acquired pneumonia (CAP) have not been conducted in every country globally. Nevertheless, important aspects regarding the frequency of pathogens encountered in different countries have been reported. Some of these are highlighted below:

- *Streptococcus pneumoniae* remains a prominent, if not the commonest, cause of CAP in the majority of countries
- Tuberculosis (TB) is a major cause of community acquired pneumonia (CAP) in TB endemic areas. It accounts for 12–21% of CAP in Hong Kong and Singapore, and 7% in India. Some studies of CAP exclude patients with *M. tuberculosis*, making direct comparisons between studies more difficult
- Gram-negative bacteria such as *Klebsiella pneumoniae* are commoner in some countries in Africa (e.g. South Africa) and the Far East (e.g. Taiwan, China) compared to Europe, accounting for 10–15% of pathogens isolated in CAP. Very high frequencies of *Staphyloccocus aureus* (42%) and *Mycoplasma pneumoniae* (36%) have been reported from Bangladesh, Pakistan and India, whereas other studies have confirmed the predominance of *S. pneumoniae*, reinforcing the importance of locally relevant data
- Legionella pneumonia has not been reported as frequently in the tropics as in European and US studies.

The possibility of TB presenting as an acute pneumonia in regions with a high prevalence of TB gives rise to particular challenges. The obvious concern is that of patients with TB being misdiagnosed as having CAP and consequently being treated with antibacterial agents that are ineffective. However, an equally important concern relates to the use of quinolones for the initial empirical treatment of CAP. (Unfortunately, some countries with high rates of penicillin-resistant pneumococcal infections where quinolones might be promoted for CAP, also happen to be areas where TB is endemic.) Such use may lead to partial symptom resolution in unrecognised TB resulting in delayed diagnosis. A further concern is the potential to select for quinolone-resistant *M. tuberculosis* strains as a result of exposure to quinolone monotherapy in these patients. Therefore, in patients from TB endemic areas presenting with CAP, pulmonary TB should be always considered and adequate microbiological evaluation for *M. tuberculosis* should be performed.

10.2.1 Melioidosis

Infection by *Burkholderia pseudomallaei* ('melioidosis') is a common cause of severe CAP in endemic areas and is notable for several reasons:

- It is only sensitive to a selected range of antibiotics and not therefore always covered by initial empirical antibiotic regimens recommended for CAP in non-endemic areas
- It is not uncommonly misidentified in microbiology laboratories in non-endemic areas, and
- It carries a particularly high mortality.

Thailand has the highest number of reported cases of melioidosis, especially north-east Thailand, followed by Malaysia, Singapore, and northern Australia. In Thailand, *Burkholderia pseudomallei* accounts for 32–55% of cases of CAP in hospitalized patients. Cases have also been reported from the Indian subcontinent and Burma. Imported cases in people returning from endemic areas usually represent recent infection. Reactivation from a latent focus is well recognized with reported latent periods extending up to many decades. However, reactivation is on the whole relatively uncommon as evident from the small number of cases diagnosed amongst the 225,000 US veterans of the Vietnam war with subclinical infection (based on positive serological testing).

Burkholderia pseudomallaei is a Gram-negative bacillus that is present as free-living saprophytes in soil and surface waters in endemic areas. It thrives in stagnant, muddy water. Infection usually occurs following percutaneous inoculation through breaks in the skin, or less commonly through inhalation of the bacteria. In endemic areas, the main recognized risk factors for melioidosis are diabetes (13 times increased risk), alcohol excess, renal disease and chronic lung disease (4 times increased risk).

10.2.2 Clinical presentations

Apart from asymptomatic infection, there is a wide spectrum of clinical presentation ranging from localised skin ulcers or abscesses, to fulminant disseminated septicaemia (45–87% mortality). Half of all cases of melioidosis present with pneumonia and half of hospitalized cases are bacteraemic. Whatever the clinical presentation, multiple abscesses are common especially in the spleen, kidney, prostate, and liver.

Patients with acute septicaemic melioidosis pneumonia present with high fevers, systemic collapse and often minimal cough or pleuritic pain. Chest radiography often reveals diffuse nodular infiltrates in both lungs which coalesce and cavitate. Not uncommonly progression is rapid and the patient may succumb within 24–48 hours despite intensive treatment.

Alternatively, some patients present with a productive cough, dyspnoea and chest radiography revealing consolidation in one or more lobes. Upper lobe involvement is common, in contrast to pneumococcal pneumonia which predominantly affects the lower lobes (Box 10.1).

> ### Box 10.1 Chest radiographic features of melioidosis
> - Upper lobe involvement—common in acute pneumonia; classically seen in chronic infection; often mistaken for TB
> - Diffuse nodular infiltrates in both lungs—in septicaemic pneumonia; progresses rapidly
> - Pleural effusions and hilar lymphadenopathy—uncommon

Patients with chronic pulmonary melioidosis present with fever, weight loss, productive cough, pleuritic chest pain, and occasionally haemoptysis. The illness is progressive over a period of months. Upper lobe infiltrates with cavitation is typical. The main differential diagnosis is pulmonary tuberculosis.

10.2.3 Diagnosis

A positive culture is the only way to achieve a definitive diagnosis of melioidosis. *B. pseudomallei* grows readily in standard blood culture media. However, laboratories in non-endemic areas may misidentify the bacteria unless alerted to the possibility of melioidosis. Serological tests do not distinguish exposure from active infection.

10.2.4 Treatment

B. pseudomallei is typically resistant to penicillin, ampicillin, first and second-generation cephalopsorins, gentamicin and tobramycin. It is generally susceptible to co-amoxiclav, ceftazidime, ceftriaxone, cefotaxime, imipenem, meropenem, piperacillin, chloramphenicol, co-trimoxazole (trimethoprim/sulfamethoxazole) and doxycycline. This susceptibility profile helps distinguish it from *Pseudomonas aeruginosa*.

Initial intensive therapy centres around the use of ceftazidime, meropenem or imipenem for a minimum of 10–14 days. Co-trimoxazole (up to 1920mg 12 hourly—double-strength dose) may be added. The benefit of combination therapy over monotherapy has not been conclusively demonstrated.

Following initial intensive therapy, prolonged eradication therapy is required to prevent subsequent relapse. A minimum 12 week course of co-trimoxazole (up to 1920mg 12 hourly—double-strength dose) is recommended, possibly in combination with doxycyline. Co-amoxiclav is recommended as an alternative to co-trimoxazole for eradication therapy in pregnancy and in children.

10.3 Pulmonary involvement with other infections from the tropics

The 3 main parasitic infections worldwide are malaria (>300 million individuals annually), schistosomiasis (>200 million infected persons) and amoebiasis (>100 million infected persons). Although pulmonary involvement is not usually the main disease manifestation of these infections, respiratory symptoms are not uncommon and may be important in establishing the initial diagnosis or in the differential diagnosis. Specific treatment of these infections is not covered in the text.

10.3.1 Malaria

Malaria as a cause of pneumonia is not fully substantiated. If it exists as a separate entity, it is very rare. Most pneumonias associated with malaria are secondary bacterial pneumonias.

- A self-limiting cough may occur in up to 36% of cases of falciparum malaria and 53% of ovale malaria
- Pulmonary oedema and ARDS is associated with severe falciparum malaria. Unlike malaria related renal failure, coagulopathy, or cerebral malaria, malaria related ARDS occurs later in the illness. It can occur following a few days of antimalarial therapy and there may be no evidence of heavy parasitaemia at the time of onset. The reason for the delayed presentation is not fully known. Cytokine damage is likely. Patients are usually gravely ill. The differential diagnosis includes hospital-acquired pneumonia.

10.3.2 Schistosomiasis

Schistosomiasis is one of 10 leading causes of morbidity among travellers and is caused by the larvae of *Schistosoma mansoni, S. haematobium* and *S. japonicum*. Over 50% of travellers on rafting tours in Africa are reported to become infected. The disease is also endemic in many countries in the Far East, e.g. China, Japan, Philippines, Thailand. The lungs are affected in both acute and chronic schistosomiasis.

- Acute schistosomiasis is a seroconversion illness experienced by non-immune visitors to endemic areas. A history of contact with infected freshwaters (e.g. swim or watersports in lakes/rivers) is common. Following exposure (incubation period of 5 weeks), patients present with fever, rigors, sweats, myalgia, weakness. A dry cough is present in 30–65%. Eosinophilia is usually present. Chest x-ray abnormalities include non-specific infiltrates and hilar lymphadenopathy. The illness is self-limiting with resolution after about 3 months
- Chronic schistosomiasis is seen mainly in residents in endemic areas. The main manifestations are related to the gastrointestinal tract. Pulmonary involvement is generally associated with

concurrent hepatosplenomegaly and portal hypertension. Eggs are released from the portal circulation to the lungs via porto-systemic collaterals. A granulomatous reaction with fibrosis is incited leading to pulmonary hypertension and cor pulmonale

- A Jarish-Herxheimer reaction comprising of cough, wheeze, eosinophilia, and chest radiographic infiltrates may occur with treatment (praziquantel is the treatment of choice).

10.3.3 **Amoebiasis**

Infection by the protozoan *Entamoeba histolytica* is described world-wide but especially in India, Southeast Asia, South America, South Africa, and parts of the Middle East. It is linked with poverty and lack of safe drinking water, and occurs predominantly in men (male to female ratio 9:1). Amoebiasis is the third leading cause of death due to parasitic infections in the world.

- Pleuropulmonary amoebiasis occurs exclusively in patients with liver abscesses
- Patients typically present with a right lower lobe lung abscess manifesting with symptoms of fever, right pleuritic chest pain, dry cough, and sometimes, haemoptysis
- Expectoration of 'anchovy-sauce' coloured sputum/pus should raise the suspicion of a hepatobronchial fistula.

10.3.4 **Less common tropical infections**

Infections that are relatively less common in endemic areas pose a diagnostic challenge to physicians in non-endemic areas. Co-infection with HIV further complicates the situation, and of course, some 'tropical infections' have a world-wide distribution, though they are commoner in the tropics. Occasionally there are specific environmental exposures that are associated with certain infections. Table 10.1 offers some 'diagnostic clues' to a few of the more prominent infections to consider in returning travellers, highlighting the relevant respiratory components.

Table 10.1 'Diagnostic clues' to infections from the tropics with pulmonary involvement		
Exposure/high incidence areas*	**Typical clinical features**	**Pathogen/infection & comments**
Contact with waters contaminated with infected urine (e.g. walk, swim in rivers). Incubation 7–10 days. Widely distributed.	Fever, chills, headache, muscle pains. Cough in 30%. Patchy alveolar changes on CXR. In severe disease, features of pulmonary haemorrhage.	Leptospirosis. Bacterial infection. Usually self-limiting. Massive pulmonary haemorrhage in severe disease. Animal reservoirs— rats, dogs, cattle, pigs.

Table 10.1 (Contd.)

CHAPTER 10 Less common infections

Exposure/high incidence areas*	Typical clinical features	Pathogen/infection & comments
Consumption of infected crustaceans (e.g. inadequately cooked crabs). Incubation 3–24 months. Far East, Africa, Central & South America.	Insidious illness. Haemoptysis, cough, chest pain. Eosinophilia. Pleural effusion and ring shadows on CXR.	Paragoniamiasis (lung fluke) Parasitic infection. 20% of patients may be asymptomatic despite infection.
Consumption of contaminated food or water. Symptoms occur when lung cyst expands or ruptures. Middle East, Australia, northern & eastern Africa, southern & western South America.	Cough, dyspnoea, chest pain, haemoptysis, expectoration of 'grapeskins'(cyst membrane) with a salty taste. May present as pneumothorax. Solitary or multiple cysts on CXR.	Echinococcosis (hydatid lung disease). Parasitic infection. Lungs are the second commonest site of infection after the liver.
Widely distributed in tropics.	Immunocompetent—Cough, wheeze, eosinophilia (Loeffler's syndrome), serpiginous urticarial eruption (larva currens). Immunocompromised—severe diarrhoea, septic shock, ARDS.	Strongyloides stercoralis. Parasitic infection. Differential diagnosis – asthma. Hyperinfection in immunocompromised. Eosinophilia may be absent. History of travel may be distant.
Contact of breached skin with contaminated soil. Inhalation of organism. Thailand, South-East Asia, China	Immunocompromised patients with AIDS—severe pneumonia.	Penicilliosis marneffei. Fungal infection. Blood culture usually positive in disseminated infection. Can behave like histoplasmosis.
Exposure to bat caves. Incubation 12–21 days. Central USA—Ohio & Mississippi areas.	Acute—Fever, cough, chest pains, arthralgia, erythema multiforme or nodosum. Patchy consolidation and hilar lymphadenopathy on CXR. Chronic—Symptoms and appearances on CXR may resemble TB or lung cancer.	Histoplasmosis. Fungal infection. 99% of infected persons in endemic areas are asymptomatic.
Contact with rodents. Incubation 3–28 days. North, Central and South America.	Fever, dyspnoea. Bilateral interstitial infiltrates on CXR.	Hantavirus pulmonary syndrome. Usually self-limiting. In severe disease, ARDS with high mortality.

*these are not exclusive geographical areas.

Further reading

Anstey N.M., Jacups S.P., Cain T., et al. (2002) Pulmonary manifestations of uncomplicated falciparum and vivax malaria: cough, small airways obstruction, impaired gas transfer, and increased pulmonary phagocytic activity. *J Infect Dis* **185**(9): 1326–34.

Chang K.C., Leung C.C., Yew W.W., et al. (2010) Newer fluoroquinolones for treating respiratory infection: do they mask tuberculosis? *Eur Respir J* **35**(3): 606–13.

Currie B.J., Fisher D.A., Howard D.M., et al. (2000) Endemic melioidosis in tropical northern Australia: a 10-year prospective study and review of the literature. *Clin Infect Dis* **31**: 981–6.

Low D.E. (2009) Fluoroquinolones for treatment of community-acquired pneumonia and tuberculosis: putting the risk of resistance into perspective. *Clinical Infectious Diseases* **48**: 1361–3.

Mabeza G.F., Macfarlane J. (2003) Pulmonary actinomycosis. *Eur Respir J* **21**(3): 545–51.

Song J.H., Oh W.S., Kang C.I., et al. Asian Network for Surveillance of Resistant Pathogens Study Group (2008) Epidemiology and clinical outcomes of community-acquired pneumonia in adult patients in Asian countries: a prospective study by the Asian network for surveillance of resistant pathogens. *Int J Antimicrob Agents* **31**(2): 107–14.

Tsang K.W and File T.M. Jr (2008) Respiratory infections unique to Asia. *Respirology* **13**: 937–49.

Udwadia Z.F (2006) Tropical respiratory diseases: in *Respiratory Infections* (1st edn) eds: Torres A., Ewig S., Mandell L., Woodhead M. Hodder Arnold.

Chapter 11

Antibiotics in respiratory tract infections

Wei Shen Lim

Key points

- Beta-lactam antibiotics include pencillins, cephalosporins, carbapanems (e.g. meropenem), and monobactams (e.g. aztreonam)
- Oral co-amoxiclav has generally higher activity than oral cephalosporins
- Only 10% of patients with a history of penicillin allergy have allergic reactions when treated with penicillin.
- The quinolone antibiotics differ in their activity against *Streptococcus pneumoniae*
- Extensive use of quinolones has been associated with increased healthcare acquired infections such as *Clostridium difficile* infections and MRSA
- In the management of pneumococcal pneumonia, low and moderate levels of penicillin-resistance are not associated with treatment failure, whereas both macrolide-resistance and quinolone-resistance are.

11.1 Introduction

Ideally, antibiotics would only be used in bacterial infections where eradication of the pathogen results in improved clinical outcome. However, in the management of respiratory tract infections, antibiotics are often prescribed on an empirical basis when the pathogen involved has not yet been identified.

Good stewardship of the use of antibiotics requires:

- Confirmation of the diagnosis as rapidly as possible
- Review of antibiotic use according to clinical status
- Use of pathogen-specific antibiotics where possible once the pathogen has been identified.

To lower the chances for the development of antibiotic resistance, rapid bacterial eradication and the elimination of resistant pathogens from colonized areas are important.

11.2 **Classes of antibiotics**

11.2.1 **Beta-lactams**

There is often confusion regarding antibiotic classes and antibiotic names, especially with regards to the beta-lactam antibiotics. All antibiotics in this class contain a cyclic amide (a β-lactam) and are further divided according to the nature of the cycle (see Table 11.1). In general, beta-lactam antibiotics are not active against *Mycoplamsa sp.*, *Legionella sp.* or *Chlamydophila sp.* Activity against other Gram-positive or Gram-negative bacteria varies according to sub-class of antibiotic.

Table 11.1 Selected properties of beta-lactam antibiotics	
Class/agent	**Properties and comments**
Penicillins (class) Benzylpenicillin	Narrow spectrum of activity, mainly Gram-positive bacteria. No activity against penicillanase-producing *Staph aureus*.
Amoxicillin	Broad activity against Gram-positive and Gram-negative bacteria. No activity against penicillanase-producing organisms.
Co-amoxiclav (amoxicillin + clavulanic acid)	Clavulanic acid extends the activity of amoxicillin to include some beta-lactamase-producing organisms. Broad activity against Gram-positive, Gram-negative and anaerobic bacteria.
Flucloxacillin	Narrow spectrum of activity, mainly Gram-positive bacteria. Predominantly used to treat meticillin-sensitive *Staph aureus*. Avoid in penicillin allergy.
Cephalosporins (class)	5–10% cross-reactivity in penicillin allergy–significance is debated.
2nd generation, e.g. cefuroxime	Broad activity against Gram-positive and Gram-negative bacteria. More activity against staphylococci compared to 3rd generation cephalosporins.
3rd generation, e.g. ceftriaxone	Broad activity against Gram-positive and Gram-negative bacteria. Some have activity against *P. aeruginosa* e.g. ceftazidime, cefotaxime.
4th generation, e.g. cefipime (unlicensed in UK)	Excellent Gram positive and Gram negative coverage including against *Pseudomonas aeruginosa*.

Table 11.1 (*Contd.*)	
Class/agent	Properties and comments
Carbapanems (class) e.g. meropenem, imipenem	Broad activity against Gram-positive and Gram-negative bacteria. Active against *Pseudomonas aeruginosa* Some cross-reactivity in penicillin allergy.
Monobactam (class) e.g. Aztreonam	Mainly only active against Gram-negative bacteria. Not active against Gram-positive bacteria or anaerobic bacteria. Not absorbed from gastrointestinal tract. Can be used in penicillin allergy, no cross-reactivity.

For most beta-lactams, a time above MIC of over 40% is required to achieve 85–100% bacteriological cure. In relation to orally administrated antibiotics, this is more confidently achieved with oral co-amoxiclav than oral cephalosporins. Of the oral cephalosporins, cefprozil (not licenced in the UK) and cefpodoxime have higher activity than cefixime, cefuroxime and cefaclor.

11.2.2 Penicillin allergy

Penicillin allergy can have an important impact on management decisions. Unfortunately, patients may be inappropriately labelled as having an allergy to penicillin. Key points to note are:

- A history of penicillin allergy is obtained from about 10% of hospitalized patients
- Only 10% of patients with a history of penicillin allergy have allergic reactions when treated with penicillin
- Aminopenicillins (e.g. ampicillin) are associated with a nonallergic rash during some viral illnesses
- A non-pruritic morbilliform rash occurring >72 hours after administration is not usually IgE mediated. A test dose of the drug may be warranted.

11.2.3 Macrolides

Macrolides bind reversibly to the 50S ribosomal subunit, thus inhibiting bacterial cell-wall synthesis. They are bacteriostatic with activity against a range of Gram-positive and Gram-negative bacteria including *Mycoplamsa sp. Chlamydophila sp.* and *Legionella sp.*

The commonly used agents are erythromycin, clarithromycin, and azithromycin. Less gastrointestinal side-effects are apparent with clarithromycin and azithromcyin compared to erythromycin. Azithromycin displays high tissue concentrations.

Macrolides interact with cytochrome p450 in the liver which may result in drug interactions.

11.2.4 **Ketolides**

A relatively new class of antibiotics is the ketolides. Telithromycin is the currently available agent. Confusingly, telithromycin is sometimes referred to as a new macrolide while other texts do not include telithromycin when referring to macrolides. Telithromycin, like the macrolides, interacts with the 50S ribosomal subunit, and also with 23S rRNA. It displays a wide range of activity against Gram-positive and Gram-negative bacteria, including *Mycoplamsa sp., Chlamydophila sp., Legionella sp.* and *Staphylococcus aureus*. It is bactericidal against *S. pneumoniae* and is active against most macrolide-resistant strains of *S. pneumoniae*.

11.2.5 **Quinolones**

Quinolones inhibit the bacterial topoisomeriases, DNA gyrase and topoisomerase IV, thus inhibiting DNA synthesis. Early agents in this class of antibiotic included nalidixic acid and norfloxacin. These were mainly active against some Gram-negative organisms and were used for the treatment of urinary tract infections. The introduction of ciprofloxacin, with activity against *P. aeruginosa*, *Staph* aureus, *Mycoplamsa sp.*, *Chlamydophila sp.* and *Legionella sp.* led to its wide use in respiratory tract infections (see Table 11.2).

Unfortunately, the extensive use of quinolones has been associated with increases in healthcare acquired infections such as *C. difficile* infections and MRSA.

Table 11.2 Selected properties of commonly used quinolones in respiratory tract infections	
Agent	**Selected properties and comments**
Ciprofloxacin	Activity against *P. aeruginosa* *Low activity* against *S. pneumoniae*.
Levofloxacin	No activity against *P. aeruginosa* *Moderate* activity against *S. pneumoniae*.
Moxifloxacin	No activity against *P. aeruginosa*. High activity against Gram-positive bacteria, including *S. pneumoniae*.
All of the above	Activity against *Staph* aureus, *Mycoplamsa sp.*, *Chlamydophila sp.* and *Legionella sp.* Good oral bioavailability. Bactericidal.

Table 11.3 Brief notes on other antibiotics commonly used in respiratory tract infections

Class/agent	Selected properties and comments
Aminoglycosides (class) e.g. gentamicin, tobramycin	Interfers with mRNA translation. Bactericidal. Active against aerobic and facultative Gram-negative bacteria. Active against *P. aeruginosa*. Can usually be dosed once daily—Cmax/MIC ratio >10 for best activity
Tetracyclines (class) e.g. tetracycline, doxycycline	Inhibits bacterial protein synthesis. Bacteriostatic. Activity against *Mycoplamsa sp.*, *Chlamydophila sp.* and *Legionella sp.* Avoid in pregnancy and young children.
Glycopeptides (class) e.g. vancomycin, teicoplanin.	Active against Gram-positive bacteria, including MRSA. Bactericidal. Used mainly for MRSA infections. Vancomycin is poorly concentrated in the lung and oral bioavailability is too low to treat systemic infections.
Oxazolidinones (class) e.g. linezolid	Active against Gram-positive bacteria, including MRSA. Bacteriostatic. Good tissue penetration, including lung tissue. Oral bioavailability of linezolid is good.
Lincosamides (class) e.g.clindamycin	Active against Gram-positive, including *S. aureus* and anaerobic bacteria. Bactericidal. Not active against *Haemophlius influenzae*. Good oral bioavailability (90%) and food does not interfere with its absorption.
Co-trimoxazole (trimethoprim-sulfamethoxazole)	Inhibits bacterial synthesis of dihydrofolic acid. Possibly bactericidal. Broad activity against Gram-positive and Gram-negative bacteria. Serious and fatal haematologic adverse reactions have been reported.
Chloramphenicol	Inhibits protein synthesis. Mainly bacteriostatic with some bactericidal activity against *H. influenzae* and *S. pneumoniae*. Activity against *Mycoplamsa sp.*, *Chlamydophila sp.* and anaerobic bacteria. Inexpensive. Used in many developing countries. Narrow therapeutic window. Severe aplastic anaemic is reported–no distinct correlation with dose/duration of treatment.

11.3 Antibiotic resistance of *Streptococcus pneumoniae*

11.3.1 Resistance to penicillin

Resistance rates of *S. pneumoniae* to penicillin vary across the world:

- Very high rates in some countries in East Asia (e.g. >70% in Vietnam and Korea)
- High rates in some European countries (e.g. 40–50% in Spain and France)
- Moderate rates in the US (<20% of bloodstream pneumococcal infections)
- Low rates in the UK and Denmark (<4%).

In addition, a high proportion (>60%) of penicillin-resistant *S. pneumoniae* strains are also resistance to other antibiotics such as erythromycin, tetracycline, clindamycin, co-trimoxazole, and chloramphenicol.

Some knowledge of local prevalence rates of antibiotic resistance to *S. pneumoniae* is important given the wide geographical variation that can occur even within countries. The spread of a few resistance clones has been the main factor contributing to the global spread of resistance. In Spain, serotypes 6, 9, 14, 19 and 23 account for 83% of penicillin-resistant *S. pneumoniae*.

Resistance to penicillin and other beta-lactams is due to alterations in penicillin-binding proteins (PBP), of which there are 6. The affinity of beta-lactam antibiotics for any particular PBP varies. Different alterations in PBPs result in different levels of penicillin resistance as well as different levels of susceptibility to other antibiotics, such as amoxicillin, cephalosporins and carbapanems. Fortunately, high level penicillin resistance (MIC $\geq$ 8µg/ml) is uncommon.

High dose oral amoxicillin will still achieve the target of >40% dosing interval above MIC for respiratory tract infections caused by *S. pneumoniae* strains with low and moderate levels of penicillin resistance (i.e. MIC up to 4µg/ml). There are some data to suggest that penicillin-resistant *S. pneumoniae* strains are less virulent than susceptible strains, giving rise to less bacteraemic disease. Certainly, non-randomized studies have not reported any significant increase in mortality in hospitalized patients treated with high dose beta-lactam antibiotics (penicillins or cephalosporins) for penicillin-resistant *S. pneumoniae* respiratory tract infections.

11.3.2 Resistance to macrolides

Resistance of *S. pneumoniae* to macrolides is mediated through 2 mechanisms:

- Target-site modification encoded by *erm*B gene. Found world-wide.

- Efflux pump—driving the drug out of the cell, encoded by *mef* A gene. Predominates in the US.

Unlike penicillin resistance in *S. pneumoniae*, macrolide-resistance resulting from either mechanism is associated with a worse outcome in patients with respiratory tract infections treated only with a macrolide. One case-control study reported that whilst taking a macrolide antibiotic, 24% of 76 patients had breakthrough bacteraemia with an erythromcyin resistant strain of *S. pneumoniae* compared to no breakthrough bacteraemias in 136 controls with erythromycin-susceptible strains.

Macrolide resistance is a more prominent problem than penicillin resistance in many parts of East Asia. For instance, rates of erythromycin resistance in Vietnam, Taiwan, Korea, Hong Kong, and China are over 70%, with very high MIC levels (>128 mg/L) reported. In contrast, the rate of erythromycin–resistance in the UK is around 9%.

Isolates of *S. pneumoniae* that express both *erm*B and *mef*A have been reported with increasing frequency in the US. Almost all of these isolates are highly resistant to multiple antibiotics including penicillin, macrolides and tetracycline. A proportion are also resistant to co-amoxiclav.

11.3.3 **Resistance to quinolones**

Resistance of *S. pneumoniae* to quinolones occurs from mutations in the *gyrA* and *parC* genes which encode for DNA gyrase and topoisomerase IV respectively. An initial mutation in either gene leads to decreased quinolone susceptibility. A subsequent mutation in the second gene leads to full resistance. Therefore emergence of resistance during treatment is most likely to develop from strains that already carry one mutation.

Understandably, previous quinolone exposure is a risk factor for quinolone-resistance. The potential for quinolones to select for mutant strains differs—in descending order: levofloxacin > moxifloxacin (least likely).

China and Hong Kong have reported high rates of quinolone resistance amongst *S. pneumoniae* isolates. Monotherapy with quinolones for infections caused by *S. pneumoniae* strains exhibiting quinolone-resistance has been associated with treatment failure.

11.3.4 **Clinical implications of antibiotic resistance in the treatment of pneumococcal respiratory tract infections**

- Infections caused by penicillin-resistant *S. pneumoniae* can usually be treated with adequate doses of penicillins and cephalosporins without clinical failure. This supports the empirical use of penicillins for presumed pneumococcal respiratory tract infections
- Macrolide resistance is associated with treatment failure. When considering monotherapy with a macrolide for pneumococcal

infection, the issue of antibiotic resistance should be taken into account

- Quinolone resistance is associated with treatment failure. Previous recent exposure (<3 months) to a quinolone is a risk factor for the development of quinolone resistance which should be considered particularly in patients with recurrent infections.

11.4 Pregnancy and the use of antibiotics

A report in 2006 reviewed 124 references relating to the use of 11 antibiotics in pregnant and lactating women. The teratogenic potential and quality of data with regards to antibiotics commonly used in respiratory tract infections are given in Table 11.4.

Exposure to tetracycline in the second and third trimesters of pregnancy has been associated with yellow-brown staining and banding of the teeth of the child and reversible growth retardation of the long bones. There are no corresponding data for doxycycline. Nevertheless, it is an FDA category D drug and is generally avoided in pregnancy when possible. Erythromycin (FDA category B) has not been significantly associated with an increased risk of malformations or other forms of foetal toxicity in human pregnancy.

Table 11.4 Teratogenic potential of some common antibiotics

Antibiotic	Quality of data	Teratogenicity risk	FDA category*
Benzylpenicillin	Good	None	B
Phenoxymethyl-penicillin	Good	None	B
Amoxicillin	Fair	Unlikely	B
Doxycycline	Fair	Unlikely	D
Ciprofloxacin	Fair	Unlikely	C
Levofloxacin	Fair	Unlikely	C
Clindamycin	Limited	Undetermined	B

*US Food and Drug Administration (FDA) Pregnancy Category:

B = animal studies do not indicate a risk to the foetus and there are no controlled human studies, or animal studies do show an adverse effect on the foetus but well controlled studies in pregnant women have failed to demonstrate a risk to the foetus.

C = studies have shown that the drug exerts animal teratogenic or embryocidal effects, but there are no controlled studies in women, or no studies are available in either animals or women.

D = positive evidence of human foetal risk exists, but benefits in certain situations may make use of the drug acceptable despite its risks.

Further reading

Centers for Disease Control and Prevention (CDC) (2008) Effects of new penicillin susceptibility breakpoints for Streptococcus pneumoniae–United States, 2006–2007. *MMWR Morb Mortal Wkly Rep.* **57**(50): 1353–5.

Lim W.S., Macfarlane J.T., Colthorpe C.L. (2003) Treatment of community-acquired lower respiratory tract infections during pregnancy. *Am J Respir Med* **2**(3): 221–233.

Lonks J.R., Garau J., Medeiros A.A. (2002) Implications of antimicrobial resistance in the empirical treatment of community-acquired respiratory tract infections: the case of macrolides. *J Antimicrob Chemother* **50**: S2:87–92. Review.

Nahum G.G., Uhl K., Kennedy D.L. (2006) Antibiotic use in pregnancy and lactation: what is and is not known about teratogenic and toxic risks. *Obstet Gynecol* **107**(5): 1120–38.

Romano A., Gaeta F., Valluzzi RL., et al. (2010) IgE-mediated hypersensitivity to cephalosporins: cross-reactivity and tolerability of penicillins, monobactams, and carbapenems. *J Allergy Clin Immunol* **126**(5): 994–9.

Yates A.B. (2008) Management of patients with a history of allergy to beta-lactam antibiotics. *Am J Med* **121**(7): 572–6.

Further reading

Centers for Disease Control and Prevention (CDC) (2005). Update to new guidelines, and updated indications for Streptococcus pneumoniae infections. Clin Infect Dis, 40(9) A, MMWR Morb Mortal Wkly Rep, 37(50), 1311–5.

DiNubile MJ, Hutchinson CE (2003). Treatment of community-acquired lower respiratory tract infections, during pregnancy. Curr Respir Infect, 31(6): 223–231.

Fekety R, Shah AB, Anderberg AA (2009). Implications of antibiotic-resistant organisms. Treatment of penicillin-resistant reduction over a ten-year resistant pneumoniae. J Am Pharm Assoc, 51(6): 65–72.

Mandell LA, Bartlett JG, Dowell SF, et al. Update on the diagnosis and treatment of acute otitis media and community-acquired pneumonia, 44(Suppl 2): 27–72.

Ramirez J, Gordon FL, et al (2003). Open-label non-comparative study in adults with community-acquired lower respiratory tract infections. J Respir Crit Care Med, 12(6): 155–161.

Whitney CG (2003). Pharmacological management of community-acquired pneumonia. A review. Arch Intern Med, 163(16): 1793–1802.

Index

Note: page numbers in *italics* refer to Figures, Tables, and Boxes.

127